WEIGHT WATCHERS

Freestyle Cookbook 2018

The Ultimate 100 Quick, Easy and Delicious Recipes
with Smart Points for Rapid Weight Loss

By Arran M. Smith

Table of Content

Introduction

Greetings readers! I want to thank you for purchasing my book. I look forward to helping you reach your weight loss goals this year and beyond.

As known to all, the weight watchers program has been known as for the function of weight loss for several decades. It can help you to form healthy habits, eating smarter, getting more exercise and losing weight.

I have participated and researched in this field for 4 years and written some experience of mine in this cookbook. The core purpose of writing this cookbook is aim to help you, my readers to lose weight and keep fit.

This book is divided into two parts. The first part is about weight watchers program, you can learn what is weight watchers program and its' some benefits. Also, you will learn the smart point and how to calculate etc. In the second part, you will see 100 delicious and easy to make weight watchers recipes, which include breakfast, appetizer, soup, snack, vegetable, dessert, and drink. You can make it whatever you wanna have.

So, what are you waiting for? Let's get started.

Chapter 1: The Weight Watchers Program

What is the Weight Watchers?

As I said before, Weight Watchers is well known for several decades, it is one of the best diet plans that can help you to lose weight and keep fit. It is not going to be as restrictive as some of the other diet plans that are out there. You are not going to have to pick whether you are allowed to eat grains or eating some fats in your diet. You will get to pick out the foods that you would like to eat, but you will be limited somewhat on the number of points, known as Smart Points in this program, that you are allowed to eat each day. This makes it a little bit healthier to follow because you will be able to choose a lot of healthy and tasty foods, you won't be stuck eating foods that are unhealthy and bad for the body or having to feel like you are deprived all the time.

Let's take a look at this program a bit more. The idea behind Weight Watchers is to make you more conscious about the food choices that you are making. Many diet plans tell you to avoid this or that and then concentrate too much on the number of calories that you are consuming. As long as you are staying in this calorie count, they promise that you are going to lose weight. The issue is that it isn't always about the number of calories that you are eating as it is about the type of calories that you consume. 100 calories of fruit are much different than the 100 calories of a cookie, and this is what the Weight Watchers diet focus on.

With the diet, you will be given a set amount of Smart Points that you are allowed to have each day, and then you can have a few more during the week when you want a cheat day or to eat out every once in a while. The number of points that you are allowed will be based on your profile. Depending on your height, current weight, and how much you would like to lose, you will be given an amount of Smart Points that you can use up each week.

Basics of the Weight Watchers Plan

Weight Loss Freestyle program is one of the best weight loss programs you can get on. It allows you to lose a lot of weight safely and effectively. While some other diet plans make a lot of promises along the way, most of them are hard to keep up or leave you feeling deprived for a long term. When it comes to Weight Watchers, you can maintain it because it is so easy and straightforward to follow. You can live an easy life while on this diet, still having a few treats and getting to eat out when you would like, but you just have to be a bit little on the choices which you make.

The Weight Watchers program is based on a points system. When you attend our first meeting or sign up online, you will be able to learn how many points you are allowed to have during the day. The points that you get will vary based on how much you want to lose, and some other factors including weight, age, height, and activity level. The point levels will change during your journey to help you adjust to any weight loss that you have and ensures that you will continue to see results along the way.

These points are going to help you along the way really. They don't tell you exactly what you have to eat, but they will help you to pick the right choices. Foods that are high in protein and lots of proper nutrients, such as vegetables, fruits, and lean meats, will be lower in points. This means that you would be able to eat more of them before you get your point values. Options that are high in bad fats, carbs, and sugars are going to be higher in points. This means that you would be able to eat fewer of them before reaching your point allowance.

Why Choose Weight Watchers?

There are many diet plans that you can choose. Some limit your carb intake while others limit the fats. Some are healthy while others are hard to maintain because they are so strict on the body. Weight Watchers is different from others because you have some options. Some of the reasons that you should choose to go with Weight Watchers instead of another program includes:

Lose more weight—overall, people who go on a program similar to Weight Watchers can lose more weight than with other options. This is because it is flexible to follow and you have that motivation and support going to the meetings each week.

Flexibility—It is flexibility when on Weight Watchers. You can enjoy the ability to pick the foods that you want to eat, You can also pick your activity levels. This makes it easier for everyone to find the path on this plan that works best for them.

Lifestyle change—Weight Watchers, is not just about losing weight. It is about making changes in your whole lifestyle that will result in healthy body. You are going to learn how to eat foods that are healthier and full of nutrition while getting rid of the foods that are causing weight gain and health issues.

You can eat out—when you are on this plan, you are allowed to eat out. It means that you can eat out with friends and family, as long as you make the right decisions for the rest of the day and don't overdo it with eating at the restaurant, you will be fine without ruining all your hard work.

Chapter 2 Understand the Smart Points

What Are the Smart Points?

With Weight Watchers, you are not necessary to kick out any of the food groups; you are just becoming more conscious about the food decisions that you make.

When you go on the Weight Watchers plan, you have to know a points system-Smart Points. This is to help you to make decisions based on your current weight and how much you would like to use in the process. The number of points can help you to make healthier food choices. Each food that you pick will have an absolute point value, and the goal is to stay within the points each day.

These points are important when it comes to the foods that you are allowed to eat on this diet plan. Rather than focusing on the calories that you are consuming, you are going to focus on the points. These points are based on the macro and micronutrients that are inside of the food that you plan to eat during the day.

When the food has a lot of excellent macro and micronutrients like protein, good carbs, and healthy vitamins, you are going to see that they contain a smaller number of points and you can eat more of them throughout the day with your diet.

On the other hand, if the items are mostly calories, sugars, and saturated fats, they rank higher when it comes to the points that you can use.

The idea behind this is that you are encouraged to eat more of the healthier foods while to ditch some of the bad foods, although some of these bad foods are allowed on occasion when you are on the diet plan.

The Calculation of Smart Points

The things you will need to compute the Smart Points of each food item you eat include the calories, saturated fat grams, sugar grams, and protein grams. You can always find these in the nutrition facts part of your food product's package.

Calculation Formula:

$$SP = \frac{C}{33} + \frac{F}{3.67} + \frac{S}{8.25} - \frac{P}{10.3}$$

(Note: C=Calories, F=Saturated Fat, S=Sugar, P=Protein)

Either roundup or down the number you get, and what you have is the Smart Points value of the food item in question.

Remember that you must have all of the components together for you to calculate the Smart Points of your meals correctly.

Simpler Version of Calculation

There is also a more straightforward way to compute the Smart Points value of a food item if you end up wanting to do it while you are outside of your home and you could not spare time to get a calculator out.

For instance, if you are in the grocery and you are checking out the nutritional value of food, you can try this more straightforward formula:

1) Begin by dividing the total calories to 100.
2) Divide the sugar content by 8. Add the result to your answer to the previous step.
3) Divide the saturated fat content by 4. Add the result to the previous effect.
4) Move the resulting decimal point one space leftward. Afterward, subtract the result to the last estimate.
5) Round up or down as necessary.

These two computation methods should give you an idea of how much Smart Points each food item you eat costs. However, you can always rely on the official list that Weight Watchers provides if you want to make sure.

If you need more specific help as regards the Smart Point allocation for a specific type of food, you can consult a Weight Watchers specialist for more help.

Chapter 3 Useful Tips When Eating Out

People eating out is a part of life. The advice is to find the best comparison you can, and guestimate of the points what the food you eating is worth in Smart Points. Note it down, enjoy your meal and don't dwell any more on the points. Don't worry about the points detract from your feed.

Try to make sensible choices with the food you have while you're out. You must know the diets rich in oil, cream, butter, and cheese are higher in Smart Point value, and other things that are baked, steamed, have salad or fruit, are lower in Smart Points, so use a bit of common sense.

With many eating places, you can look at the menu before you go out, to work out what are the best options for you. If you decide before you go out, you'll be less likely to change your mind or be swayed by other people's orders when you get there. If you know in advance that you'll be eating out, you could ensure that the other things you eat that day are quite low in points, or have saved your weekly Smart Points allowance towards this meal out.

There are no strict rules here, simply choose the foods that you like on a daily basis. As long as they are within your points range you can go ahead and eat what you like.

I wish you all the best on your weight loss journey!

Chapter 4 Breakfast Recipes

1. Delicious Fruity Quinoa Salad
(Prep Time: 5 mins, Cook Time: 15 mins/Serves: 1)

Smart points: 5

Nutritional Values Per Serving

- Calories: 195
- Saturated Fat: 4 grams
- Carbs: 13.7 grams
- Sugar: 3 grams
- Protein: 23 grams

Ingredients

- ¼ cup of quinoa
- ½ a cup of skimmed milk
- ¼ cup of olive oil
- 1 tablespoon of honey
- 1 tablespoon dressing
- 1 large mango
- 1 kiwis
- 1 cup of fresh blueberries
- 1 cup of fresh raspberries

How to cook

1. Combine the milk, the quinoa and olive oil in a small saucepan and bring it to a boil.
2. Turn the heat down to medium and cover. Cook until the quinoa has absorbed the liquid.

3. At the same time, Wash and prepare the mongo, kiwis, blueberries and raspberries, cut mango and kiwis into pieces.
4. Add the honey into the cooked quinoa.
5. Spoon the quinoa into a bowl and mixed with fresh fruit, pour the dressing on the top of salad.
6. Serve and enjoy.

2. Cheese & Ham Breakfast Casserole
(Prep Time: 20 mins, Cook Time: 1 hour /Serves: 6)

Smart points: 5

Nutritional Values Per Serving

- Calories: 168
- Saturated Fat: 7 grams
- Carbs:17 grams
- Sugar: 6 grams
- Protein: 28 grams

Ingredients

- 1 cup of liquid egg substitute
- 4 large egg whites
- 6 slices of whole wheat bread torn into pieces
- 1 cup of lean diced ham
- ½ a cup of chopped tomatoes
- 1 cup of light Swiss cheese, shredded
- 5 cups of chopped, wilted spinach
- ¼ cup of chopped roasted peppers

- ¼ cup of chopped green onions
- 1 cup of fat free buttermilk
- 2 tablespoons of Dijon mustard
- 1 tablespoon of finely chopped fresh parsley
- ½ a teaspoon of paprika
- A few Salt and pepper
- Cooking spray

How to cook

1. Preheat the oven to 375 degrees F.
2. Grease a baking dish with cooking spray.
3. In a large bowl combine the egg whites, egg substitute, mustard, buttermilk, salt, pepper and paprika and whisk to combine.
4. In a separate large bowl, combine the roasted red peppers, green onions, parsley, ham, bread, spinach and tomatoes. Toss to combine.
5. Transfer the ingredients into the baking dish and press down into the dish. Put foil over the top and bake for 45 minutes.
6. Remove the foil and sprinkle the cheese over the top, continue baking for another 15 minutes.
7. Remove from the oven and allow the casserole to cool down before serving.

3. Mushroom, Bacon and Cheese Muffin
(Prep Time: 15 mins, Cook Time: 20 mins/Serves: 12)

Smart points: 4

Nutritional Values Per Serving

- Calories: 176
- Saturated Fat: 4 grams
- Carbs: 10 grams
- Sugar: 3 grams
- Protein: 32 grams

Ingredients

- 2 cups of whole wheat flour
- 1 cup of all-purpose flour
- ½ a cup of liquid egg substitute
- 1 1/3 cups of non-fat buttermilk
- 1 cup of finely chopped green onions
- ¾ cup of diced turkey bacon, extra lean
- ½ a cup of low fat cheddar cheese, grated
- ½ a cup of finely diced mushrooms
- 1 tablespoon of baking powder
- ½ a teaspoon of baking soda
- Salt and pepper
- ½ a teaspoon of garlic powder
- 3 tablespoons of extra virgin olive oil
- 2 tablespoons of melted light butter

How to cook

1. Preheat the oven to 400 degrees F.

2. Grease a 12 cups muffin tray with cooking spray.
3. Combine the baking soda, baking powder, garlic powder, flour and salt and pepper in a large bowl. Toss to combine.
4. In a medium bowl whisk together the butter, oil, buttermilk and eggs.
5. Add the mushrooms, cheese, bacon and onions.
6. Combine the wet ingredients with the dry ingredients and stir to combine.
7. Scoop the batter into the muffin cups and bake for 20 minutes.
8. Remove from the oven and leave to cool down before serving.

4. Sandwich with Cheese
(Prep Time: 5 mins, Cook Time: 25 mins/Serves: 1)

Smart points: 5

Nutritional Values Per Serving

- Calories: 230
- Saturated Fat: 2 grams
- Carbs: 25 grams
- Sugar: 5 grams
- Protein: 33 grams

Ingredients

- 1 sandwich round
- 1/3 cup of liquid egg whites
- ½ a teaspoon of salt
- ¼ teaspoon of pepper

- 1 slice of fat free cheese of your choice
- ¼ cup of chopped spinach leaves
- 1 slice of lean deli ham
- 2 slices of fresh tomato
- 1 slice of red onion
- Cooking spray

How to cook

1. Spray a frying pan with cooking spray and heat over medium temperature.
2. Toast the sandwich round.
3. Fry the ham until the edges get crispy.
4. Arrange the ham on 1 half of the sandwich round.
5. Sauté the spinach.
6. Add the egg whites, scramble and season with salt and pepper.
7. Gather the eggs into a heap and top with cheese.
8. Cover the frying pan and allow the cheese to melt.
9. Arrange the spinach and the eggs onto the sandwich round.
10. Top with the onion and tomato and the other half of the sandwich round and serve.

5. Avocado Toast with Cherry Tomatoes
(Prep Time: 5 mins, Cook Time:10 mins/Serves: 4)

Smart points: 4

Nutritional Values Per Serving

- Calories: 168
- Saturated Fat: 10 grams
- Carbs: 16 grams
- Sugar: 5 grams
- Protein: 46 grams

Ingredients

- 4 slices of whole grain bread
- 1 large avocado
- 1 clove of minced garlic
- 1 cup of fresh sprouts
- 1 cup of halved cherry tomatoes
- The juice of ½ a lime
- Salt and pepper

How to cook

1. Slice the avocado in half, remove the stone and scoop out the flesh into a bowl.
2. Add the garlic, lime juice and salt and pepper and stir to combine.
3. Toast the bread and spread the avocado mixture over each slice.
4. Top with tomatoes and sprouts and then serve.

6. Portobello Mushrooms Eggs
(Prep Time: 5 mins, Cook Time:15 mins/Serves: 2)

Smart points: 4

Nutritional Values Per Serving

- Calories: 151
- Saturated Fat: 8 grams
- Carbs: 2 grams
- Sugar: 0 grams
- Protein: 28 grams

Ingredients

- 2 large Portobello mushrooms, stems removed
- 2 large eggs
- 4 cups of fresh baby spinach
- 1 teaspoon of olive oil
- 4 slices of bacon
- ¼ cup of Hollandaise sauce
- Salt and pepper
- Cooking spray

How to cook

1. Preheat the oven to 400 degrees.
2. Line a baking tray with parchment paper
3. Spray the mushrooms with cooking spray and season with salt and pepper.
4. Top the mushrooms with two slices of bacon and arrange on the baking tray.

5. Roast the mushrooms for 10 minutes, once cooked, remove them from the oven.
6. Heat the olive oil in a frying pan over medium temperature.
7. Sauté the spinach and the garlic.
8. Poach the eggs in a poaching pan.
9. Put the mushrooms onto plates and layer the mushrooms with spinach, egg and the Hollandaise sauce.

7.Banana Oat Strawberry Smoothie
(Prep Time: 5 minutes/Serves: 2)

Smart points: 9

Nutritional Values Per Serving

- Calories: 305
- Saturated Fat: 3.75 grams
- Carbs: 55.89 grams
- Sugar: 8.19 grams
- Protein: 26.46 grams

Ingredients

- 1 cup of almond milk, unsweetened
- 1 cup of Greek yogurt, fat free
- 2 cups of strawberries
- 2 large bananas
- ½ a cup of quick oats

How to cook

1. Blend the oats until they turn into a flour.

2. Add the rest of the ingredients and blend until smooth.
3. Pour into glasses and serve.

8. Raisin Granola with Coconut
(Prep Time: 5 mins, Cook Time: 15 mins/Serves: 12)

Smart points: 6

Nutritional Values Per Serving

- Calories: 215
- Saturated Fat: 3 grams
- Carbs: 34 grams
- Sugar: 8 grams
- Protein: 24 grams

Ingredients

- 2 cups of quick oats
- 2 cups of old fashioned oats
- 1 tablespoon of cinnamon
- 1 cup of raisins
- A pinch of salt
- ½ a cup of unsweetened shredded coconut
- 1 ½ teaspoons of vanilla
- ¼ cup of melted butter
- ¼ cup of honey

How to cook

1. Preheat the oven to 350 degrees F.
2. Combine all ingredients in a large bowl and stir to combine.
3. Arrange the granola onto a baking tray and bake for 20 minutes.

4. Once cooked, remove the granola from the oven, let it cool down and then serve with milk.

9. Blueberry Milk Pancakes
(Prep Time: 15 mins, Cook Time: 5mins/Serves: 7)

Smart points: 5

Nutritional Values Per Serving

- Calories: 205
- Saturated Fat: 2 grams
- Carbs: 31 grams
- Sugar: 4 grams
- Protein: 22 grams

Ingredients

- 1 ½ cups of whole wheat flour
- 3 teaspoons of baking powder
- 1 teaspoon of salt
- 2 tablespoons of sugar
- 1 ½ cups of skim milk
- 1 egg
- 2 tablespoons of vegetable oil
- 2 cups of blueberries
- Cooking spray

How to cook

1. Sift the dry ingredients together and set to one side.
2. In a large bowl, combine the oil, eggs and milk and whisk together thoroughly.

3. Add half of the flour ingredients and stir together thoroughly.
4. Add the remainder of the flour mixture and stir together thoroughly.
5. Add the blueberries and stir.
6. Spray a frying pan with cooking spray and heat over medium temperature.
7. Pour the batter into the frying pan and cook the pancakes for 2 minutes on both sides. They should be golden brown in color.

10. Blueberry Parfait
(Prep Time: 10 minutes/Serves: 1)

Smart points: 8

Nutritional Values Per Serving

- Calories: 278
- Saturated Fat: 3.1 grams
- Carbs: 49 grams
- Sugar: 8.8 grams
- Protein: 23.5 grams

Ingredients

- 2/3 cup of plain Greek yogurt, non fat
- 1 cup of fresh blueberries
- 1/3 cup of whole grain granola, unsweetened
- 1 tablespoon of chia seeds

How to cook

1. Layer a bowl with yogurt, granola and blueberries, top with chia seeds and serve.

Chapter 5 Main Dish Recipes

11. Feta & Spinach Greek Frittata
(Prep Time: 3 mins, Cook Time: 32 mins/Serves: 4)

Smart points: 6

Nutritional Values Per Serving

- Calories: 328
- Saturated Fat: 6 grams
- Carbs: 14 grams
- Sugar: 1 gram
- Protein: 58 grams

Ingredients

- 2 cups of fat free egg whites
- 2/3 cup of crumbled feta cheese
- 2 tablespoons of fresh dill
- Salt and pepper
- 1 diced medium onion
- 5 ounces of baby spinach
- ½ a cup of roasted red bell pepper
- 2 seeded and diced plum tomatoes
- Cooking spray

How to cook

1. Preheat the oven to 350 degrees F.
2. Combine the egg substitute, dill, feta cheese, salt and pepper and whisk together thoroughly.

3. Spray a large frying pan with cooking spray and heat it over high temperature.
4. Cook the onion for 6 minutes.
5. Add the spinach and cook until it wilts.
6. Add the tomatoes and roasted pepper and cook for another 1 minute.
7. Pour the egg mixture into the frying pan and cook for 5 minutes.
8. Put the frying pan in the oven and bake for 20 minutes.
9. Once the center has set, take the frying pan out of the oven and serve.

12. Macaroni with Cheese
(Prep Time: 25 minutes/Serves: 8)

Smart points: 6

Nutritional Values Per Serving

- Calories: 233
- Saturated Fat: 5.2 grams
- Carbs: 39 grams
- Sugar: 3 grams
- Protein: 31.3 grams

Ingredients

- 2 ½ cups of elbow macaroni
- 4 tablespoons of all purpose flour
- 2 teaspoons of dry mustard
- Salt and pepper
- 2 ¼ cups of milk, fat free

- ¼ cup of softened cream cheese, fat free
- 2 ½ cups of cheddar cheese, low fat

How to cook

1. Cook the macaroni according to the instructions on the packet.
2. In a large saucepan combine the flour, cayenne, salt, pepper, dry mustard and milk and whisk together thoroughly.
3. Add the cream cheese and bring the mixture to a boil over high heat stirring continuously.
4. Turn the heat down and allow the mixture to gently bubble until it starts to thicken and the cream cheese has melted. This should take around 2 minutes. Remove the saucepan from the cooker.
5. Add the cheddar cheese and let it melt.
6. Add the pasta and stir to coat. Divide onto plates and serve.

13. Asian Squash Spaghetti Salad
(Prep Time: 10 mins, Cook Time: 1 hour /Serves:8)

Smart points: 4

Nutritional Values Per Serving

- Calories: 158
- Saturated Fat: 2 grams
- Carbs: 12 grams
- Sugar: 0.4 grams

- Protein: 18 gram

Ingredients

- 1 spaghetti squash
- ¼ cup of sesame ginger dressing, low fat
- Salt
- 1/8 a teaspoon of dried red pepper flakes
- 1 diced red bell pepper
- ½ an English cucumber, seeded and diced
- 1 large thinly sliced scallion

How to cook

1. Preheat the oven to 375 degrees F.
2. Prick the outside of the squash with a fork, put it on a baking tray and bake for 1 hour. Flip them over half way through.
3. Once cooked, remove it from the oven and allow it to cool down before slicing.
4. Cut the squash horizontally and scoop out the pulp and the seeds.
5. Use a fork to scrape out the squash into a large bowl and allow it to cool down.
6. Drizzle the salad dressing over the top, scallion, bell pepper and pepper flakes. Toss to combine.
7. Divide onto plates and serve.

14. Avocado Tomato Onion Scramble
(Prep Time: 15 mins, Cook Time:5 mins/Serves: 4)

Smart points: 7

Nutritional Values Per Serving

- Calories: 279
- Saturated Fat: 4 grams
- Carbs: 12 grams
- Sugar: 3 grams
- Protein: 31 grams

Ingredients

- 2 teaspoons of olive oil
- 2 cups of chopped broccoli
- 1 chopped red pepper
- ½ a cup of diced onions
- 8 whisked eggs
- 1 diced tomato
- 1 chopped avocado
- Salt and pepper

How to cook

1. Heat the olive oil in a saucepan and sauté the red pepper, broccoli, and onion for 4 minutes.
2. Add the eggs and stir continuously.
3. Add the avocado and tomato and stir to combine.
4. Season with salt and pepper, divide onto plates and serve.

15. Spinach, Oregano, Sweet Potato Casserole
(Prep Time: 5 mins, Cook Time:45 mins/Serves: 4)

Smart points: 7

Nutritional Values Per Serving

- Calories: 264
- Saturated Fat: 8 grams
- Carbs: 24 grams
- Sugar: 0.7 grams
- Protein: 35 grams

Ingredients

- 2 teaspoons of olive oil
- 3 cups of sweet potato diced and peeled
- ½ a diced red onion
- ½ a teaspoon of salt
- ½ a teaspoon of garlic powder
- ½ a teaspoon of oregano
- ½ a teaspoon of pepper
- 4 cups of chopped spinach
- Cooking spray
- 8 eggs

How to cook

1. Heat the olive oil in a large saucepan over medium temperature.
2. Add the sweet potato and the onions and cook for 10 minutes. Prevent burning by adding tablespoons of water.
3. Add the oregano, garlic powder, pepper and salt.

4. Add the spinach and cook until it wilts.
5. Grease a baking tray with cooking spray and transfer the mixture onto it.
6. Whisks the eggs and pour them into the baking tray.
7. Bake for 30 minutes. Once the eggs are set, remove the baking tray from the oven divide onto plates and serve.

16. Garlic Thai Chili Chicken
(Prep Time: 10 mins, Cook Time: 40 mins/Serves: 4)

Smart points: 8

Nutritional Values Per Serving

- Calories: 296
- Saturated Fat: 6.6 grams
- Carbs: 8 grams
- Sugar: 2 grams
- Protein: 28.2 grams

Ingredients

- 1 pound of chicken breast tenders
- Cooking spray
- ¼ cup of chili garlic sauce
- 2 tablespoons of honey
- Salt and pepper
- 2 cups of chopped asparagus spears
- 1 cup of chopped onion
- 1 tablespoon of olive oil
- Cooked rice

How to cook

1. Preheat the oven to 375 degrees F.
2. Spray a baking tray with cooking spray.
3. Arrange the chicken on the baking tray and season with salt and pepper.
4. Combine the honey, chili sauce and garlic in a small bowl and whisk together thoroughly.
5. Pour the mixture over the chicken and distribute it evenly using a basing brush.
6. Add the onion and asparagus and drizzle olive oil over the top.
7. Bake for 30 minutes until the chicken is properly cooked.
8. Remove the baking tray from the oven, let it rest for 5 minutes, divide onto plates and serve.

17. Pineapple, Broccoli Pork
(Prep Time: 7 mins, Cook Time:18 mins/Serves: 4)

Smart points: 8

Nutritional Values Per Serving

- Calories: 328
- Saturated Fat: 5.3 grams
- Carbs: 22.7 grams
- Sugar: 0.5 grams
- Protein: 37.4 grams

Ingredients

- 1 pound of trimmed vealed cutlets

- Cooking spray
- ½ a cup of whole wheat breadcrumbs
- ½ a teaspoon of paprika
- ½ a teaspoon of onion powder
- Salt and pepper
- 4 teaspoons of canola oil
- The white from 1 large egg
- 4 teaspoons of cornstarch

How to cook

1. Preheat the oven to 400 degrees F.
2. Pound the veal cutlet so that it is ½ an inch thick.
3. Line a baking tray with parchment paper and grease it with cooking spray.
4. In a shallow bowl combine the breadcrumbs, onion powder, paprika, salt and pepper and the oil and stir to combine.
5. Coat the veal with corn starch.
6. Beat the egg white until it turns into a froth.
7. Dip the veal into the egg white.
8. Dip the veal into the breadcrumbs.
9. Arrange the veal cutlets onto the baking tray and bake for 18 minutes until they turn golden brown in color.
10. Remove from the oven and serve.

18. Italian Steak Rolls and Asparagus
(Prep Time:10 mins, Cook Time: 25/Serves: 4)

Smart points: 6

Nutritional Values Per Serving

- Calories: 211
- Saturated Fat: 6.6 grams
- Carbs: 7.9 grams
- Sugar: 1.2 grams
- Protein: 24.6 grams

Ingredients

- 1 pound of thinly sliced flank steak
- ¼ cup of Italian salad dressing, low fat
- 1 cup of sliced red pepper
- ½ a pound of trimmed asparagus spears
- 1 cup of sliced onion
- Cooking spray
- Salt and pepper
- Kitchen twine

How to cook

1. Preheat the oven to 350 degrees F.
2. Marinate the steak in Italian salad dressing.
3. Line a baking tray with foil.
4. Arrange the steak on the baking tray and season with salt and pepper.
5. Arrange the onion, asparagus and red bell pepper in the middle of each piece of steak.

6. Roll the steak around the vegetables and pierce with kitchen twine to secure.
7. Spray a frying pan with cooking spray and heat over medium temperature.
8. Sear the steak rolls in the frying pan
9. Arrange the steak rolls back onto the baking tray and bake for 20 minutes until the vegetables become tender and crisp and the meat is cooked through.
10. Remove the tray from the oven and let the steak rest for 5 minutes before serving.

19. Dijon Garlic Chicken
(Prep Time: 5 mins, Cook Time:20 mins/Serves:4)

Smart points: 7

Nutritional Values Per Serving

- Calories: 246
- Saturated Fat: 6.8 grams
- Carbs: 5.1 grams
- Sugar: 2.1 grams
- Protein: 26.3 grams

Ingredients

- 4 lean beef steaks
- Cooking spray
- Salt and pepper
- ½ a teaspoon of onion powder
- ½ a teaspoon of oregano

- 1 cup of sliced leeks
- ½ a cup of dry red wine
- 1 cup of beef stock
- ¼ cup of gorgonzola cheese crumbles

How to cook

1. Spray a frying pan with cooking spray and heat over medium temperature.
2. Season the steaks with oregano, onion powder, salt and pepper.
3. Sear the steaks in the frying pan, remove onto a plate and set to one side.
4. Cook the leeks for 3 minutes.
5. Add the red wine and cook for another 3 minutes.
6. Add the beef stock and put the steak back in the frying pan.
7. Turn the heat down to low and continue to cook for 10 minutes.
8. Divide the steak and the sauce onto plates, top with the gorgonzola and serve.

20. Grilled Oregano Sesame Salmon Kebabs
(Prep Time:10 mins, Cook Time:10 mins/Serves: 2)

Smart points: 7

Nutritional Values Per Serving

- Calories: 267
- Saturated Fat: 8 grams
- Carbs: 7 grams
- Sugar: 0.5 grams

- Protein: 35 grams

Ingredients

- ½ a teaspoon of ground cumin
- 1 tablespoon of chopped fresh oregano
- ¼ teaspoon of red pepper flakes
- 1 teaspoon of sesame seeds
- 1 sliced lemon
- Salt
- Cooking spray, olive oil
- 8 bamboo skewers, soaked for 1 hour in water

How to cook

1. Preheat the grill to 395 degrees F and spray the grates with cooking spray.
2. In a small bowl, combine the oregano, sesame, red pepper and cumin.
3. Thread the salmon onto the skewers with the lemon in between.
4. Grill the salmon for 10 minutes until it turns opaque.
5. Remove from the grill and serve.

21. Grilled Chicken Raisin Salad
(Prep Time: 30 minutes/Serves:4)

Smart points: 6

Nutritional Values Per Serving

- Calories: 222
- Saturated Fat: 5.4 grams
- Carbs: 26.9 grams
- Sugar: 2 grams
- Protein: 25.0 grams

Ingredients

- ¼ cup of low fat mayonnaise
- 1 teaspoon of curry powder
- 2 teaspoons of water
- 1 pound of cooked chopped lemon herb rotisserie chicken
- ¾ cup of chopped apple
- 1/3 cup of diced celery
- 3 tablespoons of raisins
- 1/8 teaspoon of salt

How to cook

1. Combine the water, curry powder and mayonnaise in a medium sized bowl and whisk to combine.
2. Add the apple. Raisins, celery, chicken and salt and toss to combine.
3. Serve with bread or alone.

22. Parsley, Cilantro, with Salsa
(Prep Time: 25 mins, Cook Time: 5 mins/Serves: 4)

Smart points: 4

Nutritional Values Per Serving

- Calories: 184
- Saturated Fat: 2.0 grams
- Carbs: 7.6 grams
- Sugar: 1.4 grams
- Protein: 25 grams

Ingredients

- 4 ounces of boneless, trimmed pork loin chops
- Cooking spray
- 1/3 cup of salsa
- 2 tablespoons of freshly squeezed lime juice
- ¼ cup of chopped fresh parsley or cilantro

How to cook

1. Flatten the pork chops out on a flat surface.
2. Spray a large frying pan with cooking spray and heat over high temperature.
3. Cook the pork chops on each side for 1 minute until they become medium brown in color. Turn the heat down to low.
4. In a small bowl combine the lime and the salsa and whisk together thoroughly.
5. Pour the salsa mix over the pork chops and simmer for 10 minutes.

6. Divide onto plates, garnish with parsley or cilantro and serve.

23. Broccoli Slaw & Turkey Cheeseburger
(Prep Time: 15 minutes/Serves: 10)

Smart points: 8

Nutritional Values Per Serving

- Calories: 318
- Saturated Fat: 8 grams
- Carbs: 22.7 grams
- Sugar: 0.8 grams
- Protein: 38.3 grams

Ingredients

- 2 ½ pounds of lean ground turkey
- 3 cups of broccoli slaw
- 1 1/3 cups of grated carrots
- ½ a cup of blue cheese dressing
- 2 cloves of grated garlic
- ½ a cup of whole wheat seasoned breadcrumbs
- 1 tablespoon of grated red onion
- Salt and pepper
- ½ a cup of hot sauce
- 10 slices of low fat cheddar cheese
- Cooking spray
- 10 burger buns, whole wheat

How to cook

1. In a large bowl combine the turkey, hot sauce, pepper, salt, garlic, onion, carrots, breadcrumbs and turkey. Stir together thoroughly and then mold them into 10 patties.
2. In a separate bowl combine the blue cheese dressing and broccoli slaw.
3. Spray a frying pan with cooking spray and heat over a high temperature.
4. Cook the patties 2 at a time until they become golden brown in color.
5. Toast the burger buns.
6. Place a patty on top of each bun, layer with a slice of cheese and broccoli slaw and serve.

24. Sesame Ginger Chicken
(Prep Time:15 minutes, Cook Time: 20 mins/Serves:4)

Smart points: 6

Nutritional Values Per Serving

- Calories: 210
- Saturated Fat: 7.5 grams
- Carbs: 8.9 grams
- Sugar: 1.3 grams
- Protein: 25.9 grams

Ingredients

- 1 pound of ground beef
- 1 thinly sliced leek

- 2 cloves of minced garlic
- 1 teaspoon of fresh ginger
- 1 tablespoon of red curry paste
- 1 ½ cups of canned tomato sauce
- 1 teaspoon of lime zest
- 1 tablespoon of coconut aminos
- ½ a cup of canned light coconut milk
- 2 teaspoons of lime juice

How to cook

1. Heat a frying pan and brown the beef.
2. Add the red curry paste, canned tomato, ginger, garlic, and leek and stir to combine. Bring to a boil for 10 minutes and then reduce to a simmer.
3. Add the coconut milk and the coconut aminos and simmer for a further 10 minutes.
4. Add the lime zest and the lime juice, stir to combine and serve.

25. Whitefish Lemon Dijon
(Prep Time:5 mins, Cook Time:25 mins/Serves:4)

Smart points: 1

Nutritional Values Per Serving

- Calories: 99
- Saturated Fat: 1.0 grams
- Carbs: 0.4 grams
- Sugar: 0.3 grams

- Protein: 23 grams

Ingredients

- 1 pound of whitefish fillets
- Cooking spray
- 2 tablespoons of Dijon mustard
- 1 teaspoon of prepared horseradish
- 1 tablespoon of fresh lemon juice
- Salt and pepper
- 1 sliced lemon

How to cook

1. Preheat the oven to 450 degrees F.
2. Spray a baking tray with cooking spray.
3. Combine the lemon juice, horseradish and Dijon mustard in a small bowl, stir together thoroughly.
4. Brush the fish fillets with the Dijon mixture and season with salt and pepper.
5. Arrange the fish on the baking tray, lay the lemon slices over the top of the fish.
6. Bake the fish for 15 minutes, remove from the oven and serve.

26. Chili Ginger Salmon
(Prep Time: 15 minutes/Serves: 5)

Smart points: 5

Nutritional Values Per Serving

- Calories: 233
- Saturated Fat: 5 grams
- Carbs: 8 gram
- Sugar: 3 grams
- Protein: 37 grams

Ingredients

- 3 ounces of skinless coho chicken fillets
- Salt and pepper
- ¼ teaspoon of smoked paprika
- ¼ teaspoon of ground ginger
- ¾ teaspoon of ground cumin
- 2 ½ teaspoons of olive oil
- 2 ½ teaspoons of chili powder
- Cooking spray

How to cook

1. Combine all of the dry spices in a bowl.
2. Grease the salmon with cooking spray.
3. Dip the salmon into the spice mixture.
4. Heat the olive oil in a frying pan over medium heat and cook the salmon for 5 minutes per side.
5. Remove from the pan and serve.

27. Asparagus, Cherry Tomato Salad
(Prep Time: 10 minutes/Serves: 2)

Smart points: 5

Nutritional Values Per Serving

- Calories: 164
- Saturated Fat: 6.5 grams
- Carbs: 14 grams
- Sugar: 0.4 grams
- Protein: 27 grams

Ingredients

- 8 ounces of chopped cooked lobster
- 3 ½ cups of steamed, chopped asparagus
- 2 tablespoons of lemon juice
- 4 teaspoons of extra virgin olive oil
- Salt and pepper
- ½ a cup of halved cherry tomatoes
- 1 chopped basil leaf
- 2 tablespoons of diced red onion

How to cook

1. In a small bowl, whisk together the oil, lemon juice and salt and pepper.
2. Combine the rest of the ingredients in a salad bowl.
3. Pour the dressing over the top and toss to combine.
4. Divide onto plates and serve.

28: Salmon with Coconut
(Prep Time: 20 minutes/Serves: 5)

Smart points: 5

Nutritional Values Per Serving

- Calories: 287
- Saturated Fat: 10 grams
- Carbs: 13 gram
- Sugar: 2.5 grams
- Protein: 39 grams

Ingredients

- 30 ounces of boneless, skinless salmon
- 1/3 cup of shredded unsweetened coconut
- 2 whisked egg whites
- Salt and pepper
- Cooking spray

How to cook

1. Preheat the oven to 395 degrees F.
2. Use the salt and pepper to season the salmon.
3. Dip the salmon into the egg white and them into the coconut.
4. Grease a baking tray with cooking spray.
5. Arrange the salmon on the tray and bake for 15 minutes.
6. Remove from the oven and serve.

29. Honey Baked Shrimp
(Prep Time: 15 minutes/Serves: 4)

Smart points: 3

Nutritional Values Per Serving

- Calories: 123
- Saturated Fat: 2.0 grams
- Carbs: 6.0 grams
- Sugar: 3 grams
- Protein: 16 grams

Ingredients

- ½ a pound of tuna
- 1 cup of quartered artichoke hearts
- 1 cup of chopped red bell pepper
- 1 cup of quartered cherry tomatoes
- 1 tablespoon of lemon juice
- 2 tablespoons of olive oil
- Salt and pepper
- ½ a teaspoon of oregano
- ½ a cup of chopped fresh parsley

How to cook

1. Combine the tomatoes, red bell pepper, artichoke and tuna.
2. Add the olive oil, lemon juice, oregano, salt, pepper and parsley and toss to combine.
3. Divide onto plates and serve.

30. Garlic, Parsley Shrimp Pasta
(Prep Time: 15 minutes/Serves: 1)

Smart points: 8

Nutritional Values Per Serving

- Calories: 315
- Saturated Fat: 6 grams
- Carbs: 16.7 grams
- Sugar: 0.8 grams
- Protein: 35.1 grams

Ingredients

- ¼ cup of chopped onions
- 2 chopped cloves of garlic
- 1 teaspoon of olive oil
- 2 tablespoons of white wine
- ½ a cup of cooked shrimp
- Fresh parsley
- 1 cup of cooked whole wheat pasta
- 1 tablespoon of grated parmesan cheese
- Black pepper

How to cook

1. Heat the olive oil in a frying pan.
2. Saute the garlic and onions.
3. Add the wine and turn the heat down.
4. Add the shrimp and parsley.
5. Add the pasta and stir to combine.
6. Add the pepper.
7. Add the cheese and stir to combine.
8. Transfer onto a place and eat.

Chapter 6 Appetizer Recipes

31. Chicken Bites Wrapped in Bacon
(Prep Time: 5 mins, Cook Time:25 mins/Serves: 10)

Smart points: 2

Nutritional Values Per Serving

- Calories: 70.1
- Saturated Fat: 2 grams
- Carbs: 0 gram
- Sugar: 0 grams
- Protein: 12.1 grams

Ingredients

- 3 pieces of skinless, boneless chicken breast cut into small chunks. (about 30 pieces)
- 10 pieces of bacon, sliced into thirds

How to cook

1. Preheat the oven to 395 degrees F.
2. Wrap a slice of bacon around each piece of chicken and pierce with a toothpick to secure.
3. Arrange the chicken bites on a baking tray.
4. Bake for 25 minutes until browned.
5. Remove from the oven and serve.

32. Artichoke and Spinach Dip
(Prep Time: 5 mins, Cook Time: 25 mins/Serves: 15)

Smart points: 3

- Calories: 73
- Saturated Fat: 4.5 grams
- Carbs: 3.5 gram
- Sugar: 1 gram
- Protein: 5 grams

Ingredients

- 13.75 ounces of drained artichoke hearts in water
- 10 ounces of thawed frozen spinach, water squeezed out
- ¼ cup of shallots
- 1 clove of garlic
- ½ a cup of Greek yogurt, fat free
- 4 ounces of shredded mozzarella cheese
- Salt and pepper
- Olive oil cooking spray
- Tortilla chips

How to cook

- Preheat the oven to 375 degrees F.
- Chop the shallots, garlic and artichoke hearts in a food processor.
- Add all the ingredients into a medium sized bowl and stir to combine.
- Transfer the ingredients into an oven proof dish and bake for 25 minutes.
- Remove from the oven and serve.

33. Coconut Shrimp
(Prep Time:5 mins, Cook Time: 25 mins/Serves: 8)

Smart points: 5

Nutritional Values Per Serving

- Calories: 161.5
- Saturated Fat: 3.5 grams
- Carbs: 22 grams
- Sugar: 2 grams
- Protein: 10 grams

Ingredients for the shrimp

- 24 large shrimp, deveined and peeled
- ½ a cup of sweetened, shredded coconut
- 1 tablespoon of sweetened, shredded coconut
- ½ a cup of panko crumbs
- 1 tablespoon of panko crumbs
- 2 tablespoons of all purpose flour
- 1 large egg
- A pinch of salt
- Cooking spray

Ingredients for the dipping sauce

- ½ a cup of apricot preserves
- 1 tablespoons of rice wine vinegar
- ¾ teaspoons of crushed red pepper flakes

How to cook

1. Preheat the oven to 425 degrees F.
2. Grease a baking tray with cooking spray.

3. In a small bowl, combine the panko crumbs and coconut flakes.
4. Pour the flour onto a small plate.
5. Whisk the egg in a small bowl.
6. Season the shrimp with salt.
7. Dip the shrimp into the flour, then into the egg and then into the coconut crumb mixture.
8. Arrange the shrimp onto the baking tray and spray them with cooking spray.
9. Bake the shrimp for 10 minutes, flip them over and bake for a further 10 minutes.
10. To make the dipping sauce, combine all ingredients into a small bowl and stir together thoroughly.
11. Once cooked, remove the shrimp from the oven and serve with the dipping sauce.

34. Bacon and Spinach Stuffed Mushrooms
(Prep Time: 10 mins, Cook Time:35 mins/Serves: 10)

Smart points: 1

Nutritional Values Per Serving

- Calories: 34.5
- Saturated Fat: 1.5 grams
- Carbs: 3 grams
- Sugar: 1 gram
- Protein: 3 grams

Ingredients

- 1 packet of mushrooms, stems removed
- 2 cloves of garlic thinly sliced

- 4 cups of fresh baby spinach
- 4 slices of bacon, center cut
- 1 teaspoon of olive oil
- ¼ cup of bread crumbs, Italian seasoned
- 2 tablespoons of Parmesan cheese, shredded
- Cooking spray

How to cook

1. Preheat the oven to 400 degrees F.
2. Line a baking tray with foil and grease it with cooking spray.
3. Mince the stems from the mushrooms.
4. Heat a medium sized frying pan and cook the spinach for 2 minutes until it starts to wilt.
5. Remove the spinach from the frying pan, squeeze out the excess water, chop finely and ser to one side.
6. Cook the bacon, remove it from the pan, chop coarsely and set to one side.
7. Add olive oil to the frying pan and sauté the garlic for 2 minutes.
8. Add the minced mushroom stems and sauté for another 2 minutes.
9. In a large bowl combine the parmesan cheese, bread crumbs, bacon, spinach and minced mushroom stems. Stir to combine.
10. Season the mushroom caps with salt and fill them with the spinach mixture.
11. Arrange them in a baking dish, spray with cooking oil and bake for 20 minutes.
12. Remove from the oven and serve.

35. Tomato, Avocado and Black Bean Salad
(Prep Time: 15 mins/Serves: 10)

Smart points: 4

Nutritional Values Per Serving

- Calories: 127
- Saturated Fat: 5.5 grams
- Carbs: 16 grams
- Sugar: 2.5 grams
- Protein: 15 grams

Ingredients

- 1 seedless cucumber, diced and peeled
- 2 ripe medium sized tomatoes, diced
- 2 diced haas avocados
- 1 can of black beans drained and rinsed
- 2 tablespoons of minced red onions
- 2 tablespoons of minced cilantro
- The juice of 2 limes
- Salt and pepper

How to cook

1. Combine all ingredients in a large bowl and season with salt and pepper.
2. Divide into dishes and serve.

36. Parmesan Creamy Spinach Dip
(Prep Time: 10 mins/Serves: 8)

Smart points: 2

Nutritional Values Per Serving

- Calories: 89.4
- Saturated Fat: 6.2 grams
- Carbs: 23.3 grams
- Sugar: 0.9 grams
- Protein: 23 grams

Ingredients

- 10 ounces of freshly chopped spinach
- ½ a cup of light sour cream
- 5 tablespoons of light mayonnaise
- 1/3 cup of Parmigiano Reggiano
- ¼ cup of chopped scallions
- Fresh pepper

How to cook

1. Transfer all the ingredients into a medium sized bowl and stir to combine. Refrigerate for 1 hour and serve with Ritz crackers.

37. Mustard Devilled Eggs
(Prep Time: 20 minutes/Serves: 4)

Smart points: 3

Nutritional Values Per Serving

- Calories: 96.8
- Saturated Fat: 5 grams
- Carbs: 8 grams
- Sugar: 0 grams
- Protein: 16 grams

Ingredients

- 4 large hard boiled eggs, peeled
- 2 tablespoons of Hellmann's light mayonnaise
- 1 teaspoon of Dijon mustard
- Paprika
- Salt and pepper
- 2 tablespoons of chopped chives

How to cook

1. Cut the eggs in half lengthways.
2. Take the yolks out and put them into a bowl.
3. Add mustard, mayonnaise, salt and pepper and stir together thoroughly.
4. Spoon the yolk mixture into the holes where the yolks were.
5. Garnish with chives and serve.

38. Edamame Hummus
(Prep Time: 10 minutes/Serves: 6)

Smart points: 3

Nutritional Values Per Serving

- Calories: 97.4
- Saturated Fat: 3.7 grams
- Carbs: 17.2 grams
- Sugar: 3.8 grams
- Protein: 14 grams

Ingredients

- 1 ½ cups of edamame, shelled and cooked
- 2 tablespoons of tahini paste
- ¼ cup of water
- 1 teaspoon of lemon zest
- The juice of one 1 lemon
- 1 clove of crushed garlic
- Salt and pepper
- 2 teaspoons of olive oil
- White and black sesame seeds for garnish
- Carrots/Cucumber/Celery sticks for garnish

How to cook

1. Blend the garlic, lemon zest, lemon juice, water, tahini, soy beans, olive oil, salt and pepper in a food processor.
2. Transfer the blended mixture into a bowl, top with the rest of the oil, garnish with the sesame seeds and serve with vegetable sticks of your choice.

39. Ceviche Shrimp Cocktail
(Prep Time: 20 minutes/Serves: 9)

Smart points: 3

Nutritional Values Per Serving

- Calories: 100
- Saturated Fat: 4 grams
- Carbs: 5 grams
- Sugar: 2 grams
- Protein: 11 grams

Ingredients

- ¼ cup of chopped red onion
- The juice of 2 small limes
- 1 teaspoon of olive oil
- 1 pound of large shrimp, cooked, deveined and peeled
- 1 hass avocado, diced
- 1 diced tomato
- 1 cup of English cucumber diced
- 1 serrano pepper, minced and seeds removed
- 1 tablespoons of chopped cilantro
- Chopped cilantro for garnish
- Salt and pepper
- 1 lime sliced into wedges
- 2 ¼ cups of shredded iceberg lettuce

How to cook

1. Combine the olive oil, lime juice, red onion, salt and pepper in a small bowl. Allow the mixture to marinate for 5 minutes.
2. Combine the Serrano pepper, cucumber, tomato, avocado and shrimp in a large bowl. Season with salt, pepper and cilantro. Toss to combine.
3. Line 9 martini glasses with shredded lettuce, top with the shrimp salad, garnish with cilantro and serve with 1 wedge of lime.

40. Picante Roja Salsa
(Prep Time: 15 minutes/Serves: 6)

Smart points: 1

Nutritional Values Per Serving

- Calories: 22.5
- Saturated Fat: 1 grams
- Carbs: 3.5 grams
- Sugar: 0.8 grams
- Protein: 1.8 grams

Ingredients

- 3 medium tomatoes, quartered and cored
- 1 roasted jalapeño, stem removed
- 3 small cloves of garlic
- 2 tablespoons of cilantro
- 4 tablespoons of water
- 1 teaspoon of olive oil
- Salt
- Tacos

How to cook

1. Add the water, cilantro, garlic, jalapeno and tomatoes to a food processor and blend until smooth.
2. Heat the oil in a frying pan and pour in the blended mixture. Season with salt and simmer for 25 minutes stirring occasionally.
3. Pour into small bowls and serve with tacos.

Chapter 7 Vegetarian Recipes

41. Blue Cheese and Pear Salad
(Prep Time: 20 minutes/Serves: 8)

Smart points: 4

Nutritional Values Per Serving

- Calories: 152
- Saturated Fat: 4 grams
- Carbs: 13 grams
- Sugar: 3 grams
- Protein: 20 grams

Ingredients

- 10 cups of mixed baby greens
- 3 medium pears, thinly sliced and cored
- ¼ cup of pear nectar
- 2 tablespoons of walnut oil
- 2 tablespoons of white wine vinegar
- 1 teaspoon of Dijon mustard
- 1/8 teaspoon of ground ginger
- 1/8 teaspoon of ground black pepper
- 1 teaspoon of honey
- ½ a cup of toasted broken walnuts
- ½ a cup of crumbled blue cheese of your choice

How to cook

1. Combine the mixed baby greens and pear slices in a large salad bowl and toss to combine.

2. For the dressing, combine the pepper, ginger, mustard, vinegar, honey, oil and nectar in a screw top jar. Screw the top on and shake to combine.
3. Drizzle the dressing over the salad and toss to coat.
4. Divide the salad among plates and top with walnuts and crumbled blue cheese.

42. Dates, Apple and Kale Salad
(Prep Time: 20 minutes/Serves: 6)

Smart points: 4

Nutritional Values Per Serving

- Calories: 144
- Saturated Fat: 5.9 grams
- Carbs: 17.8 grams
- Sugar: 3.2 grams
- Protein: 22.3 grams

Ingredients

- 3 tablespoons of fresh lemon juice
- 1 tablespoon of extra virgin olive oil
- Kosher salt
- 1 bunch of kale, ribs discarded, and thinly chopped
- ¼ cup of dates, thinly sliced
- 1 honeycrisp apple, sliced into small chunks
- ¼ cup of toasted slivered almonds
- 2 tablespoons of dried cranberries

- 1 ounce of finely grated pecorino cheese
- Ground black pepper

How to cook

1. In a large bowl, whisk together the olive oil, lemon juice and ¼ teaspoon of salt.
2. Put the kale into the bowl and toss to coat, leave it to soak for 10 minutes.
3. Add the cheese, cranberries, almonds, apples and dates to the kale, season with salt and pepper and toss to combine.

43. Baked Potato with Cottage Cheese & Salsa
(Prep Time: 10 minutes/Serves: 1)

Smart points: 8

Nutritional Values Per Serving

- Calories: 289
- Saturated Fat: 2.5 grams
- Carbs: 46.5 grams
- Sugar: 4.3 grams
- Protein: 21.2 grams

Ingredients

- 1 large potato
- ½ a cup of low fat cottage cheese
- 1/3 cup of salsa
- Salt and pepper

How to cook

1. Wash the potato and prick it all over with a fork.
2. Microwave on full power for 5 minutes or until it becomes soft.
3. Remove the potato from the microwave and slice it open lengthwise.
4. Season with salt and pepper, break up the insides with a fork.
5. Add the cottage cheese and then top with the salsa.

44. Beans with Cauliflower Rice
(Prep Time: 20 minutes/Serves: 2)

Smart points: 8

Nutritional Values Per Serving

- Calories: 288
- Saturated Fat: 8 grams
- Carbs: 46 grams
- Sugar: 4 grams
- Protein: 36 grams

Ingredients

- ½ a medium head of cauliflower, core and leaves removed
- 1 tablespoon of olive oil
- 1 can of black beans
- 1 teaspoon of chili powder
- ½ an avocado, sliced into chunks
- 1 chopped plum tomato
- 2 chopped green onions

- 1 handful of fresh cilantro leaves
- 2 lime wedges

How to cook

1. Blend the cauliflower into rice.
2. Heat the oil in a medium frying pan and add the cauliflower. Stir and cover for 5 minutes.
3. Add the beans and chili powder to the cauliflower and stir to combine.
4. Flavor with salt and pepper.
5. Divide onto plates and top with cilantro, onion, tomato, avocado and a squirt of lime juice.

45. Black Bean & Cheese Nachos
(Prep Time: 30 minutes/Serves: 4)

Smart points: 6

Nutritional Values Per Serving

- Calories: 222
- Saturated Fat: 2 grams
- Carbs: 36 grams
- Sugar: 6 grams
- Protein: 18 grams

Ingredients

- Low fat tortilla chips
- 1 cup of grated cheese of your choice
- 1 can of rinsed and drained black beans

- 2 chopped plum tomatoes
- 2 thinly sliced scallions
- 1 seeded and diced jalapeno pepper
- 2 tablespoons of fresh cilantro, chopped
- Lime wedges to serve
- Cooking spray

How to cook

1. Preheat the oven to 400 degrees F.
2. Line a baking tray with foil and grease it with cooking spray.
3. Lay out the tortilla chips on the baking tray.
4. Top evenly with cheese, beans, tomatoes, jalapeno and scallions.
5. Bake for 20 minutes.
6. Take the tray out of the oven, sprinkle with cilantro and serve with lime wedges.

46. Mushroom, Tomato, Zucchini Skillet
(Prep Time: 40 minutes/Serves:6)

Smart points: 1

Nutritional Values Per Serving

- Calories: 65
- Saturated Fat: 2 grams
- Carbs: 4 grams
- Sugar: 1 gram
- Protein: 14 gram

Ingredients

- 1 tablespoon of olive oil
- 1 medium zucchini sliced into ¼ inch thick pieces
- 1 yellow medium summer squash sliced into ¼ inch thick pieces
- 1 cup of fresh mushrooms, sliced
- 1 cup of cherry tomatoes cut in halves
- 1 chopped green onion
- ½ a teaspoon of garlic salt

How to cook

1. Heat the oil in a large frying pan over a high temperature.
2. Add the mushrooms, yellow squash and zucchini and cook for 5 minutes stirring continuously. The vegetables should become tender and crisp.
3. Add the green onion, tomatoes and salt and cook for a further 4 minutes.
4. Divide onto plates and serve.

47.Sugar Cucumber Salad
(Prep Time: 10 minutes/Serves: 2)

Smart points: 2

Nutritional Values Per Serving

- Calories: 56
- Saturated Fat: 1 grams
- Carbs: 9 grams
- Sugar: 4 grams
- Protein: 5 grams

Ingredients

- 3 tablespoons of rice vinegar
- 2 teaspoons of sugar
- A pinch of salt
- 1 cucumber thinly sliced

How to cook

1. Combine the sweetener, vinegar and salt in a large bowl and stir together thoroughly.
2. Put the cucumber slices in the vinegar mix and stir to combine.
3. Divide onto plates and serve.

48. Yogurt Sauce with Grilled Eggplant
(Prep Time: 20 minutes/Serves: 6)

Smart points: 3

Nutritional Values Per Serving

- Calories: 86
- Saturated Fat: 1.3 grams
- Carbs: 6.8 grams
- Sugar: 3.3 grams
- Protein: 4 grams

Ingredients

- ¾ cup of plain Greek yogurt, fat-free
- 2 tablespoons of water

- ¾ teaspoons of kosher salt
- ¼ teaspoon of ground cumin
- ¼ teaspoon of finely minced garlic
- ¼ teaspoon of paprika
- 3 baby eggplants sliced lengthwise
- Cooking spray

How to cook

1. Preheat the grill to 395 degrees F.
2. Combine the paprika, garlic, cumin, salt, water and yogurt and whisk together thoroughly.
3. Spray the eggplant with cooking spray and sprinkle with salt.
4. Grill the eggplant for 10 minutes until it is lightly charred.
5. Arrange on plates and drizzle the yogurt sauce over the top.

49. Apple Yogurt Bowl
(Prep Time: 10 minutes/Serves: 4)

Smart points: 5

Nutritional Values Per Serving

- Calories: 158
- Saturated Fat: 2 grams
- Carbs: 30 grams
- Sugar: 1 gram
- Protein: 5 grams

Ingredients

- 1 cup of sweetened applesauce
- Ground nutmeg
- ½ a cup of granola with raisins, low fat
- 1 1/3 cup of Greek vanilla yogurt, low fat

How to cook

1. Combine a dash of nutmeg and the applesauce in a small bowl and stir together thoroughly.
2. Put 1 tablespoon of granola into 4 small bowls.
3. Layer with yogurt and then applesauce.
4. Sprinkle the granola over the top and serve.

50. Strawberry and Peanut Butter Wrap
(Prep Time: 10 minutes/Serves: 1)

Smart points: 8

Nutritional Values Per Serving

- Calories: 224
- Saturated Fat: 9.2 grams
- Carbs: 47 grams
- Sugar: 5 grams
- Protein: 21 grams

Ingredients

- 1 flatout flatbread
- 1 tablespoon of peanut butter
- 2 teaspoons of all-fruit spread
- 2 hulled strawberries, sliced
- ½ a banana cut lengthwise
- 1 tablespoon of granola without raisins, low fat

How to cook

1. Spread the peanut butter over the flatbread.
2. Spread the fruit spread over the rounded end.
3. Layer with granola, banana and strawberries.
4. Roll together, slice in half and eat.

Chapter 8 Soup Recipes

51. Cheesy Broccoli Soup
(Prep Time: 10 minutes/Serves: 8)

Smart Points: 4

Nutritional Values Per Serving

- Calories: 134
- Saturated Fat: 0.2 grams
- Carbs: 17 grams
- Sugar: 2 grams
- Protein: 5 grams

Ingredients

- 2 cans of chicken broth
- 2 packets of frozen broccoli
- 1 can of tomatoes
- 8 ounces of low fat Velveeta cheese

How to cook

1. Combine the chicken broth, frozen broccoli and tomatoes into a saucepan. Stir together thoroughly and boil for 8 minutes.
2. Add the cheese and stir to combine.
3. Divide into bowls and

52. Chicken Egg Drop Soup
(Prep Time: 10 minutes/Serves: 4)

Smart Points: 6

Nutritional Values Per Serving

- Calories: 212
- Saturated Fat: 5 grams
- Carbs: 17 grams
- Sugar: 4 grams
- Protein: 27 grams

Ingredients

- 4 cups of chicken broth, low sodium
- ½ a teaspoon of soy sauce
- ½ a cup of chopped chicken breast, cooked
- ½ a cup of frozen green peas
- ¼ cup of thinly sliced green onion
- 1 lightly beaten egg

How to cook

1. Combine the soy sauce and chicken broth in a large saucepan and bring it to boil over high heat.
2. Add the onion, peas and chicken and continue to boil.
3. Remove the saucepan from the cooker and add the egg. Allow the egg to set for 1 minute and then stir gently.
4. Divide into bowls and serve.

53. Vegetable Soup
(Prep Time: 20 minutes: Serves: 6)

Smart Points: 4

Nutritional Values Per Serving

- Calories: 182
- Saturated Fat: 0.7 grams
- Carbs: 12 grams
- Sugar: 0.4 grams
- Protein: 16.3 grams

Ingredients

- 1 can of diced tomatoes
- 1 can of corn
- 1 can of ready to serve minestrone soup
- 1 can of mixed vegetables
- 1 can of rinsed black beans

How to cook

1. Combine all the ingredients in a saucepan and heat.
2. Divide into bowls and serve.

54: Cabbage Soup
(Prep Time: 32 minutes/Serves: 6-8)

Smart Points: 6

Nutritional Values Per Serving

- Calories: 253
- Saturated Fat: 0.3 grams
- Carbs: 51 grams
- Sugar: 0.7 grams
- Protein: 17 grams

Ingredients

- 2 cloves of minced garlic
- 1 tablespoon of tomato paste
- 2 cups of chopped cabbage
- ½ a yellow onion, chopped
- ½ a chopped carrot
- ½ a cup of green beans
- ½ a cup of chopped zucchini
- ½ a teaspoon of basil
- ½ a teaspoon of oregano
- Salt and pepper
- Cooking spray

How to cook

1. Spray a large saucepan with cooking spray.
2. Put the saucepan on the cooker and sauté the garlic, carrots and onions for 5 minutes.
3. Add the green beans, cabbage, tomato paste, oregano, basil, and salt and pepper. Simmer for 10 minutes until the vegetables become tender.
4. Add the zucchini and simmer for a further 5 minutes.
5. Divide into bowls and serve.

55. Cheesy Chilli Pepper Soup
(Prep Time: 45 minutes/Serves: 6)

Smart Points: 5

Nutritional Values Per Serving

- Calories: 203
- Saturated Fat: 4 grams
- Carbs: 19 grams
- Sugar: 3 grams
- Protein: 23 grams

Ingredients

- 3 cans of chicken broth
- 2 bags of frozen broccoli
- 1 can of tomatoes
- 1 green chilli pepper
- 10 ounces of low fat Velveeta cheese

How to cook

1. Cut the green chilli pepper into small piece.
2. Combine the tomatoes, chilis pepper, broccoli and chicken broth in a large saucepan and simmer for 25 minutes until the vegetables become tender.
3. Slice the Velveeta into cubes, add it to the soup and let it simmer until the cheese melts.
4. Stir to combine, divide into bowls and serve.

56. Mexican Taco Turkey Soup
(Prep Time: 70 minutes/Serves: 10)

Smart Points: 6

Nutritional Values Per Serving

- Calories: 246
- Saturated Fat: 1 gram
- Carbs: 40 grams
- Sugar: 5 grams
- Protein: 21 grams

Ingredients

- 1 pound of ground turkey breast
- 1 chopped large onion
- 1 ¼ ounce of ranch dressing
- 1 ¼ ounce packet of taco seasoning
- 1 can of pinto beans
- 1 can of hot chili beans
- 1 can of whole kernel corn
- 1 can of Mexican flavour stewed tomatoes
- 1 can of stewed tomatoes

How to cook

- In a large saucepan, brown the meat and the onions.
- Add the taco seasoning and ranch dressing and stir to combine.
- Add both cans of stewed tomatoes, corn, chili beans, and pinto beans, stir to combine and simmer for 1 hour.
- Divide into bowls and serve.

57. Cauliflower Soup
(Prep Time: 35 minutes/Serves: 10)

Smart Points: 2

Nutritional Values Per Serving

- Calories: 68
- Saturated Fat: 1 gram
- Carbs: 10 grams
- Sugar: 3 grams
- Protein: 6 grams

Ingredients

- 6 cups of water
- 5 cup of diced cauliflower
- 2 cups of diced carrots
- ½ a cup of diced onion
- 1 teaspoon of dried oregano
- 1 teaspoon of dried basil
- 4 chicken stock cubes
- Salt and pepper

How to cook

1. Combine all of the ingredient apart from the salt and pepper in a large saucepan.
2. Cover and let the ingredients simmer for 20 minutes until the vegetables become tender.
3. Drain the liquid and reserve it.
4. Transfer the vegetables into a food processor and puree.
5. Pour the pureed vegetables back into the saucepan with the liquid.
6. Add the salt and pepper and stir to combine. Continue to heat for a further 5 minutes.
7. Divide into bowls and serve.

58. Tortilla Vegetable Soup
(Prep Time: 35 minutes/Serves: 9)

Smart Points: 1

Nutritional Values Per Serving

- Calories: 52
- Saturated Fat: 0.2 grams
- Carbs: 11 grams
- Sugar: 2 grams
- Protein: 7 grams

Ingredients

- 1 cup of chopped onion
- 2 cloves of chopped garlic
- 3 chopped green onions
- 1 can of diced tomatoes
- 4 cups of chicken broth, low fat
- 1/3 cup of salsa
- ½ a chopped red pepper
- ½ a chopped green onion
- 3 chopped stalks of celery
- 1/3 cup of fresh cilantro
- ½ a teaspoon of cumin
- ½ a teaspoon of chili powder
- ½ a teaspoon of basil
- 4 tablespoons of fat free sour cream
- 4 tablespoons of flour

How to cook

1. In a large saucepan, simmer the green onions, garlic and onions.

2. Add the rest of the ingredients and simmer until the vegetables become tender.
3. Divide into bowls and serve.

59. Cheesy Bacon & Potato Soup
(Prep Time: 35 minutes/Serves: 12)

Smart Points: 4

Nutritional Values Per Serving

- Calories: 159
- Saturated Fat: 2 grams
- Carbs: 25 grams
- Sugar: 3 grams
- Protein: 16 grams

Ingredients

- 4 cans of chicken broth, fat free
- 3 pounds of peeled, diced potatoes
- ½ a diced onion
- 4 slices of bacon, cooked and crumbled
- 8 ounces of Velveeta cheese, low fat
- ¼ cup of sour cream, fat free
- 2 tablespoons of flour
- 3 tablespoons of water

How to cook

1 In a large saucepan combine the potatoes and the broth and cook for 20 minutes.

2   In a frying pan sauté the onions and add them to the potatoes.
3   In a large bowl, combine the flour, whisk together thoroughly and set to one side.
4   Add the sour cream and the cheese to the potatoes and stir to combine.
5   Add the flour and water mix and stir to combine.
6   Divide into bowls, top with the crumbled bacon and serve.

60. Chicken and Greek Orzo Soup
(Prep Time: 40 minutes/Serves: 4)

Smart Points: 6

Nutritional Values Per Serving

- Calories: 245
- Saturated Fat: 5 grams
- Carbs: 21.25 grams
- Sugar: 1.5 grams
- Protein: 34 grams

Ingredients

- 6 cups of chicken broth, low fat and low sodium
- 1 teaspoon of finely chopped fresh dill
- ½ a cup of uncooked orzo
- 4 large eggs
- 1/3 cup of lemon juice
- 1 cup of shredded carrots

- Salt and pepper
- 8 ounces of roasted chicken breast, chopped

How to cook

1. In a large saucepan, combine the dill and the broth and bring it to a boil.
2. Add the orzo and turn the heat down to low, simmer for 5 minutes and take the pan off the cooker.
3. In a food processor combine 1 cup of broth, the eggs and the lemon juice.
4. Add the chicken, carrot and salt and pepper to the pan, stir to combine and simmer for 5 minutes on medium heat.
5. Turn the heat down to low, add the egg mixture and stir to combine.
6. Divide into bowls and serve.

Chapter 9 Sandwich Recipes

61. Ice Cream Sandwich
(Prep Time: 1 minutes/Serves: 1 serving)

Smart points: 6

Nutritional Values Per Serving

- Calories: 153
- Saturated Fat: 3 grams
- Carbs: 25.8 grams
- Sugar: 4 grams
- Protein: 1.6 grams

Ingredients

- 1 tablespoon of light whipped cream
- 1 piece of honey graham cracker

How to cook

1. Break the graham cracker in half
2. Spread the whipped cream on top of one piece of cracker.
3. Place the other piece of cracker on top and press it down.
4. Put the sandwich in a Ziploc bag and freeze until ready to eat.

62. Bacon Lettuce & Tomato
(Prep Time: 6 minutes/Serves: 1 serving)

Smart points: 4

Nutritional Values Per Serving

- Calories: 167
- Saturated Fat: 4 grams
- Carbs: 28 grams
- Sugar: 3 grams
- Protein: 25 grams

Ingredients

- 3 slices of bacon, center cut
- 2 slices of whole grain bread, light
- 1 tablespoon of low fat mayonnaise
- ¼ cup of lettuce
- 2 thickly cut slices of tomato
- Salt and pepper

How to cook

1. Heat a large frying pan over medium temperature.
2. Fry the bacon until it becomes crispy, this should take around 5 minutes.
3. Remove the bacon from the frying pan and drain it on paper towels.
4. Lightly toast the bread and each slice with mayonnaise.
5. Top with bacon, tomato and lettuce.
6. Season with salt and pepper and then top with the other slice of toast.
7. Cut in half and eat.

63. Cristo Monte Sandwich
(Prep Time: 18 minutes/Serves: 4)

Smart points: 8

Nutritional Values Per Serving

- Calories: 289
- Saturated Fat: 6 grams
- Carbs: 25 grams
- Sugar: 4 grams
- Protein: 29 grams

Ingredients

- 1 large egg
- 1 egg white
- ½ a cup of non fat milk
- 4 teaspoons of Dijon mustard
- 8 slices of whole wheat bread
- 4 ounces of thinly sliced cheese of your choice
- 4 ounces of low fat chicken or turkey breast, skinless and sliced
- Cooking spray

How to cook

1. In a large bowl combine the milk, egg and the egg white and whisk together thoroughly.
2. Spread the mustard over 4 slices of bread.
3. Layer with meat and then the cheese and top with the rest of the bread. Lightly press together.

4. Spray a large frying pan with cooking spray and heat over medium temperature.
5. Dip the sandwiches into the egg mixture and then put it into the frying pan.
6. Use a spatula to press down on the sandwich and cook on both sides until lightly brown, this should take approximately 4 minutes.

64. Tuna Salad Sandwich
(Prep Time: 10 minutes/Serves: 4)

Smart points: 5

Nutritional Values Per Serving

- Calories: 137
- Saturated Fat: 5 grams
- Carbs: 1 gram
- Sugar: 1 grams
- Protein: 20 grams

Ingredients

- 1 can of white tuna in water, drained
- ½ a cup of finely chopped celery
- 2 tablespoons of chopped fresh parsley
- 2 tablespoons of reduced calorie mayonnaise
- ½ a teaspoon of Dijon mustard
- 8 slices of whole wheat bread

- Salt and pepper

How to cook

1. In a medium sized bowl, combine the parsley, tuna, celery, mustard, mayonnaise and salt and pepper. Stir together thoroughly.
2. Spread the tuna mixture over 4 slices of the bread.
3. Top with the remaining bread, cut in half and serve.

65. Crab Quesadillas
(Prep Time: 20 minutes/Serves: 4)

Smart points: 9

Nutritional Values Per Serving

- Calories: 290
- Saturated Fat: 9 grams
- Carbs: 39 grams
- Sugar: 3 grams
- Protein: 26 grams

Ingredients

- 8 ounces of imitation crabmeat
- ½ a cup of shredded cheddar cheese
- 1 can of diced green chili
- ¼ cup of chopped tomatoes
- 2 tablespoons of chopped green bell peppers
- 4 tortillas
- Cooking spray

How to cook

1. Preheat the oven to 420 degrees F.
2. Combine the bell peppers, tomatoes, chili, cheese, and crabmeat and stir to combine.
3. Spray one side of a tortilla with the cooking spray.
4. Flip over the tortilla, spread ¼ of the crab meat into it and fold the tortilla in half.
5. Repeat with the rest of the tortillas and arrange them onto a baking sheet.
6. Put them in the oven and bake on one side for 10 minutes, turn them over and bake for a further 5 minutes.
7. Remove from the oven and serve.

66. Egg Salad Sandwich
(Prep Time: 20 minutes/Serves: 4)

Smart points: 2

Nutritional Values Per Serving

- Calories: 106
- Saturated Fat: 2 grams
- Carbs: 1 gram
- Sugar: 0 grams
- Protein: 18 grams

Ingredients

- 4 large hard boiled eggs, sliced
- The whites from 2 large hard boiled eggs, sliced
- 2 tablespoons of chopped fresh chives

- 2 tablespoons of mayonnaise, reduced calorie
- ½ a teaspoon of Dijon mustard
- Salt and pepper
- Dill
- 8 slices of whole wheat bread

How to cook

1. Combine the 4 hard boiled eggs, hard boiled egg whites, dill, mustard, mayonnaise and salt and pepper into a large bowl. Stir together thoroughly.
2. Spread the egg salad over 4 slices of bread and then press the other slices on top. Cut in half and serve.

67. Chicken Salad Sandwich
(Prep Time: 20 minutes/Serves: 4)

Smart points: 4

Nutritional Values Per Serving

- Calories: 195
- Saturated Fat: 2 grams
- Carbs: 3 grams
- Sugar: 1 gram
- Protein: 25 grams

Ingredients

- 1 pound of cooked skinless, boneless chicken breast sliced into cubes
- ½ a cup of finely diced celery

- 1/3 cup of finely diced dill
- ¼ cup of low calorie mayonnaise
- 2 tablespoons of low fat sour cream
- 2 tablespoons of chopped fresh parsley
- 1 teaspoon of Dijon mustard
- 1 teaspoon of fresh lemon juice
- Salt and pepper
- 8 slices of whole wheat bread

How to cook

1. In a large bowl combine the chicken, pickles, celery, mayonnaise, sour cream, lemon juice, mustard, parsley, and salt and pepper. Stir together thoroughly.
2. Spread the chicken salad over four slices of bread, top with the rest of the bread. Slice in half and serve.

68. Reuben Grilled Sandwich
(Prep Time: 16 minutes/Serves: 1 serving)

Smart points: 8

Nutritional Values Per Serving

- Calories: 311
- Saturated Fat: 3 grams
- Carbs: 30.5 grams
- Sugar: 3.5 grams
- Protein: 26 grams

Ingredients

- 2 slices of thin rye bread
- 2 ounces of sliced corned beef
- 1 slice of low fat Swiss cheese
- 1 tablespoon of Thousand Island Dressing, fat free
- ¼ cup of sauerkraut
- Cooking spray

How to cook

1. Spread the Thousand Island Dressing on both slices of the bread.
2. Spray a large frying pan with the cooking spray and heat over a medium temperature.
3. Put the corned beef into the frying pan and cook for 2 minutes.
4. Add the sauerkraut and cook for another 2 minutes.
5. Remove the sauerkraut and the corned beef from the pan, cover and set to one side.
6. Spray the frying pan again with cooking spray and place the rye bread into the pan dressing side up.
7. Top with the corned beef, sauerkraut and cheese.
8. Top with the other slice of bread with the dressing facing downwards.
9. Press down with a spatula and cook for 2 minutes. Flip the sandwich over and cook for another 2 minutes.
10. Remove from the frying pan and serve.

69. Portobello Lettuce & Tomato
(Prep Time: 20 minutes/Serves: 4)

Smart points: 5

Nutritional Values Per Serving

- Calories: 148
- Saturated Fat: 3 grams
- Carbs: 32 grams
- Sugar: 4 grams
- Protein: 7 grams

Ingredients

- 2 large Portobello mushrooms cut into strips
- 1 large sliced tomato
- 4 lettuce leaves
- 8 slices of whole wheat bread
- 2 tablespoons of light mayonnaise
- 1 tablespoon of coconut oil
- ¼ cup of maple syrup
- 3 ounces of liquid smoke
- Salt

How to cook

1. In a large bowl, combine the salt, maple syrup and the smoke and stir to combine.
2. Soak the mushroom strips in the maple syrup mixture for 15 minutes.
3. Heat the oil in a large frying pan, cook the mushrooms for 3 minutes until they are brown and crispy.
4. Spread the mayo over 4 slices of bread and top with the lettuce, tomato and mushrooms. Top with the rest of the bread, cut into halves and serve.

70. Goat Cheese and Red Pepper Roasted Wrap
(Prep Time: 10 minutes/Serves: 1 serving)

Smart points: 7

Nutritional Values Per Serving

- Calories: 236
- Saturated Fat: 7 grams
- Carbs: 31 grams
- Sugar: 5 grams
- Protein: 28 grams

Ingredients

- Lavash whole wheat bread, 1 sheet
- 1 ounce of goat cheese
- 1 roasted red bell pepper
- 4 basil leaves
- Red onion, a few slices
- 1 handful of fresh greens

How to cook

1. Preheat the Panini press.
2. Spread the goat cheese over the bread.
3. Top with the rest of the ingredients, fold the sides in and roll into a wrap.
4. Place the sandwich into the Panini press and toast for 2-4 minutes.

Chapter 10 Snack Recipes

71. Baked Plantain
(Prep Time: 40 minutes/Serves: 2)

Smart points: 5

Nutritional Values Per Serving

- Calories: 184
- Saturated Fat: 0.5 grams
- Carbs: 47 grams
- Sugar: 2 grams
- Protein: 8 grams

Ingredients

- 2 ripe medium sized plantains, thinly sliced
- Olive oil cooking spray
- Salt

How to cook

1. Preheat the oven to 395 degrees F.
2. Line a baking tray with parchment paper and spray with cooking spray.
3. Arrange the plantain onto the baking tray and sprinkle with salt.
4. Bake for 35 minutes, flipping halfway through.
5. They will be crispy and golden when cooked.

72. Sweet Potato Fritters
(Prep Time: 45 minutes/Serves: 4)

Smart points: 4

Nutritional Values Per Serving

- Calories: 103
- Saturated Fat: 4 grams
- Carbs: 14 grams
- Sugar: 2 grams
- Protein: 7 grams

Ingredients

- 2 large medium sweet potatoes, peeled
- ½ a cup of liquid egg whites
- ¼ cup of parmesan cheese, grated
- 1 teaspoon of onion powder
- ½ a teaspoon of rosemary
- ½ a teaspoon of thyme
- Salt and pepper
- Cooking spray

How to cook

1. Preheat the oven to 395 degrees F.
2. Line a baking tray with parchment paper and grease with cooking spray.
3. Grate the sweet potatoes into a medium sized bowl and use a cheesecloth to squeeze out excess water.
4. Add the rest of the ingredients to the bowl and stir to combine.

5. Scoop out the potato mixture onto the baking tray and use a spatula to flatten them out.
6. Bake the potatoes for 30 minutes, flip over after 15 minutes.
7. The potatoes are ready to serve once they are crisp and brown.

73. Cheese and Pepperoni Roll-ups
(Prep Time: 32 minutes/Serves: 8)

Smart points: 5

Nutritional Values Per Serving

- Calories: 216
- Saturated Fat: 6 grams
- Carbs: 25 grams
- Sugar: 2 grams
- Protein: 6 grams

Ingredients

- 1 packet of pizza dough, whole wheat
- 1 packet of turkey pepperoni
- 8 sticks of string cheese, light, sliced in half
- 2 tablespoons of light butter
- 1 teaspoon of garlic powder
- 1 teaspoon of Italian seasoning
- Marinara sauce
- Flour
- Cooking spray

How to cook

1. Preheat the oven to 375 degrees F.
2. Line a baking tray with parchment paper and grease it with cooking spray.
3. Dust a work surface with flour and roll the pizza dough out into a ¼ inch rectangle.
4. Cut 16 triangles out of the rectangle.
5. Arrange 3 slices of pepperoni on the wide part of each triangle.
6. Arrange a cheese stick on top of the pepperoni and roll them up.
7. Arrange the roll-ups on the baking tray seam side down.
8. Bake for 12 minutes.
9. Put the butter into a small bowl and melt it for 30 seconds in the microwave.
10. Add the Italian seasoning and the garlic powder and whisk to combine.
11. Brush the roll ups with the melted butter mix.
12. Serve with marinara sauce.

74. Chipotle Crispy Potato Skins

(Prep Time: 30 minutes/Serves: 8)

Smart points: 2

Nutritional Values Per Serving

- Calories: 57.3
- Saturated Fat: 2 grams
- Carbs: 5.8 grams
- Sugar: 0.2 grams
- Protein: 4 grams

Ingredients

- 4 large potatoes, cooked and cut lengthwise in quarters
- Olive oil cooking spray
- 1 teaspoon of chili powder
- ¼ teaspoon of hot turkey bacon, extra lean
- ¾ cups of cheddar cheese, low fat
- 2 diced medium tomatoes
- 3 finely chopped medium scallions
- ¾ cup of low fat sour cream

How to cook

1. Preheat the oven to 425 degrees F.
2. Scoop the flesh out of the potatoes, leaving a thin layer.
3. Whisk together the hot pepper sauce and chilli powder in a small bowl.
4. Spray the potato wedges with the cooking spray and arrange them on a non-stick baking tray.
5. Top with the cheese and bacon and bake for 15 minutes.
6. Garnish with scallions and tomatoes and serve with sour cream.

75. Jalapeno Poppers
(Prep Time: 30 minutes/Serves: 4)

Smart points: 4

Nutritional Values Per Serving

- Calories: 140
- Saturated Fat: 3 grams
- Carbs: 6 grams
- Sugar: 3 grams
- Protein: 15 grams

Ingredients

- Cooking spray
- 2 ounces of light cream cheese
- ½ a cup of low fat shredded cheese
- 1 tablespoon of mayonnaise, fat free
- 8 small jalapeno peppers
- ¼ cup of egg substitute, fat free
- 1 cup of Fiber One Cereal
- Salt and pepper
- 1 teaspoon of garlic powder
- 1 teaspoon of onion powder
- 16 slices of turkey bacon, extra lean

How to cook

1. Preheat the oven to 350 degrees F.
2. Grease a baking tray with cooking spray

3. Combine the mayonnaise, cheddar cheese, and cream cheese in a medium sized bowl and whisk together thoroughly.
4. Cut the jalapenos in half lengthwise and take the seeds out. (do this with rubber gloves on)
5. Scoop the cream cheese mixture into the jalapenos.
6. Pour the egg substitute into a small bowl.
7. Grind the fiber One Cereal into a breadcrumb consistency into a separate small bowl.
8. Add onion powder, garlic powder, salt and pepper into the fiber One Cereal and toss to combine.
9. Dip the jalapenos into the egg substitute and then into the fiber One Cereal.
10. Wrap a slice of bacon around each jalapeno and arrange them on the cooking tray.
11. Bake for 30 minutes.
12. Remove from the oven and serve.

76. Buffalo Chicken Wings
(Prep Time: 30 minutes/Serves: 4)

Smart points: 4

Nutritional Values Per Serving

- Calories: 150
- Saturated Fat: 4 grams
- Carbs: 3 grams
- Sugar: 2 grams
- Protein: 22 grams

Ingredients

- Olive oil cooking spray
- 12 ounces of skinless chicken wings
- 1 ¼ ounces of Taco seasoning mix of your choice
- 1 cup of red hot sauce of your choice
- ½ a cup of sour cream, fat free
- 2 tablespoons of crumbled blue cheese
- 2 tablespoons of skimmed milk, fat free
- 4 celery sticks, medium, sliced into 2 inch pieces

How to cook

1. Preheat the oven to 400 degrees F.
2. Grease a baking tray with cooking spray.
3. Tip the taco seasoning out onto a plate.
4. Pour the hot sauce into a small bowl.
5. Dip the chicken wings into the hot sauce.
6. Roll the chicken wings into the taco seasoning.
7. Arrange the chicken wings onto the baking tray and bake for 20 minutes.
8. In a small bowl, whisk together the milk, cheese and sour cream.
9. Serve the chicken wings with the celery and dip.

77. Apple Slices With Peanut Butter
(Prep Time: 5 minutes/Serves: 4)

Smart points: 7

Nutritional Values Per Serving

- Calories: 208
- Saturated Fat: 5 grams
- Carbs: 30 grams
- Sugar: 6 grams
- Protein: 12 grams

Ingredients

- 2 large apples
- ½ a cup of reconstituted powdered peanut butter
- ¼ cup of chocolate and white chips
- ¼ cup of slivered pecans and almonds

How to cook

1. Remove the core of the apple with a pairing knife or an apple corer.
2. Slice thick rings out of the apples.
3. Spread peanut butter over the apple slices.
4. Top with the nuts and chips

78. Cantaloupe Bowl Filled with Yogurt
(Prep Time: 5 minutes/Serves: 1 serving)

Smart points: 3

Nutritional Values Per Serving

- Calories: 146
- Saturated Fat: 1.5 grams
- Carbs: 15.1 grams
- Sugar: 1.5 grams
- Protein: 21 grams

Ingredients

- ½ a cantaloupe
- 6 ounces of Greek yogurt, non-fat
- 1 tablespoon of fresh raspberries
- 1 tablespoon of fresh blueberries
- 1 teaspoon of raw pepita seeds

How to cook

1. Scoop the seeds out from the middle of the cantaloupe.
2. Fill the hole with the Greek yogurt
3. Top with the berries and seeds.

79. Oat Banana Protein Balls
(Prep Time: 20 minutes/Serves: 12)

Smart points: 1

Nutritional Values Per Serving

- Calories: 47
- Saturated Fat: 0.7 grams
- Carbs: 8.0 grams
- Sugar: 1.2 grams
- Protein: 8 grams

Ingredients

- 85 grams of rolled oats
- 1 scoop of vanilla protein powder
- 1 large banana

How to cook

1. Blend the protein powder and the rolled oats.
2. Add the banana and continue to blend.
3. Scoop out the mixture, break up and mold into 12 balls and serve.

80. Cinnamon Cocoa Covered Chickpeas
(Prep Time: 45 minutes/Serves: 4)

Smart points: 6

Nutritional Values Per Serving

- Calories: 144
- Saturated Fat: 12 grams
- Carbs: 21.9 grams
- Sugar: 5.0 grams
- Protein: 23 grams

Ingredients

- 420 grams of chickpeas
- 2 teaspoons of olive oil
- 2 tablespoons of cocoa powder
- 3 teaspoons of coconut sugar
- ½ a teaspoon of cinnamon
- 1/8 teaspoon of salt

How to cook

1. Preheat the oven to 395 degrees F.
2. Line a baking tray with parchment paper.
3. Rinse and drain the chickpeas in a colander and dry them off on a towel.
4. Transfer the chickpeas into a large bowl, add the oil, cinnamon, coconut sugar, cocoa powder and salt and stir to combine.
5. Pour the chickpeas out onto the baking tray and roast them for 15 minutes.
6. Turn the oven off and leave the oven door slightly open for 15 minutes before removing the chickpeas and serving.

Chapter 11 Dessert Recipes

81. Lemon Gelatin Dessert
(Prep Time: 15 minutes/Serves: 3)

Smart points: 1

Nutritional Values Per Serving

- Calories: 31
- Saturated Fat: 1 grams
- Carbs: 12 gram
- Sugar: 3 grams
- Protein: 5 grams

Ingredients

- 1 packet of vanilla cook and serve pudding mix, sugar free
- 2 cups of water
- 1 packet of sugar free gelatin mix
- 1 whipped topping, fat-free

How to cook

1. Combine the water and the pudding mixture in a saucepan and stir to combine.
2. Bring the mixture to a boil while stirring constantly.
3. Slowly add the gelatine mixture and continue to stir.
4. Pour into bowls and leave them to set for 1 hour in the refrigerator.
5. Top with the whipped topping and serve.

82. Limoncello Fruit Salad
(Prep Time: 20 minutes/Serves: 6)

Smart points: 1

Nutritional Values Per Serving

- Calories: 28
- Saturated Fat: 2 grams
- Carbs: 3 grams
- Sugar: 4 grams
- Protein: 7 grams

Ingredients

- 7 ounces of Greek yogurt
- 1/3 cup of good bottled lemon curd
- 1 tablespoon of honey
- ¼ teaspoon of pure vanilla extract
- 2 cups of sliced strawberries
- 1 cup of raspberries
- 1 cup of blueberries
- 2 tablespoons of sugar
- 3 tablespoons of limoncello
- 1 sliced banana
- 1 fresh mint springs

How to cook

1. In a large bowl, combine the vanilla, honey, lemon curd and yogurt and whisk together thoroughly.
2. In another large bowl, combine the limoncello, sugar, blueberries, raspberries and strawberries and toss to combine.
3. Add the banana to the mixture, and toss to combine.
4. Divide the fruit into bowls, top with the lemon yogurt and serve.

83. Grape-Blackberry Sundaes
(Prep Time: 15 minutes/Serves: 4)

Smart points: 1

Nutritional Values Per Serving

- Calories: 25
- Saturated Fat: 1.5 grams
- Carbs: 4 grams
- Sugar: 5 grams
- Protein: 8 grams

Ingredients

- ¾ cup of blackberries
- ¾ cup of seedless red grapes
- 1/3 cup of sugar
- 2 teaspoons of water
- 2 cups of vanilla ice-cream

How to cook

1. Combine the blackberries, grapes, sugar and water in a small saucepan and cook over medium temperature for 10 minutes.
2. Use a slotted spoon to remove the fruit, place it in a bowl and continue to simmer the liquid for another 2 minutes until it starts to turn into a syrup.
3. Put the fruit back into the syrup and stir to combine.
4. Divide the vanilla ice-cream into 4 bowls, top with the fruit and the syrup and serve.

84. Apple Caramel Salad
(Prep Time: 1 hour 15 minutes/Serves: 8)

Smart points: 2

Nutritional Values Per Serving

- Calories: 72.2
- Saturated Fat: 0.2 grams
- Carbs: 19.1 gram
- Sugar: 3.1 grams
- Protein: 6 grams

Ingredients

- 1 container of cool whip, fat free
- 4 large apples
- 1 can of pineapple tidbits
- 1 packet of instant butterscotch pudding mix, fat free
- ¼ cup of chopped peanuts

How to cook

1. Slice the apples into small pieces and put them into a large bowl.
2. Add the rest of the ingredients to the bowl and stir to combine.
3. Put the mixture in the fridge to chill for 1 hour.
4. Divide into bowls and serve.

85. Crisp Berry Pudding
(Prep Time: 45 minutes/Serves: 6)

Smart points: 3

Nutritional Values Per Serving

- Calories: 121.6
- Saturated Fat: 1.5 grams
- Carbs: 22 grams
- Sugar: 2.3 grams
- Protein: 12 grams

Ingredients for the fruit

- 1 bag of frozen mixed berries
- 1 bag of sugar free cook an serve pudding mix
- 1 teaspoon of cinnamon
- 1 teaspoon of nutmeg
- 1 cup of milk, non fat

Ingredients for the crisp

- 1 ½ cups of old fashioned oats
- ½ a cup of Splenda sugar substitute
- 8 ounces of plain yogurt, fat free
- 1 teaspoon of almond extract
- Cooking spray

How to cook

1. Preheat the oven to 395 degrees F.
2. Grease a baking tray with cooking spray.
3. Put the fruit ingredients into the baking tray and stir to combine.
4. In a large bowl, combine the ingredients for the crisp and stir to combine.

5. Spread the crisp over the berry mixture and bake for 45 minutes.

86. Crunch Chocolate Bars
(Prep Time: 10 minutes/Serves: 24)

Smart points: 5

Nutritional Values Per Serving

- Calories: 108
- Saturated Fat: 5 grams
- Carbs: 18.3 gram
- Sugar: 4 grams
- Protein: 1 gram

Ingredients

- 6 cups of crisp rice cereal, chocolate flavor
- 1 ½ tablespoons of margarine
- 1 ½ tablespoons of peanut butter, reduced fat
- 8 ounces of large marshmallows
- 1/3 cup of low fat semisweet chocolate morsel
- Cooking spray

How to cook

1. Grease a baking tray with cooking spray.
2. Put the rice cereal into a large bowl.
3. Combine the margarine, peanut butter, and marshmallows in a saucepan. Cook over medium heat while stirring continuously.
4. Drizzle the marshmallow mixture on top of the cereal and stir to coat.
5. Add the low fat chocolate morsels and stir to combine.

6. Spoon the mixture into the prepared pan, spread out and press down with a spatula.
7. Slice into 24 bars and serve.

87. Shortcake Strawberry Kabobs
(Prep Time: 13 minutes/Serves: 4)

Smart points: 3

Nutritional Values Per Serving

- Calories: 77.7
- Saturated Fat: 3 grams
- Carbs: 9.5 gram
- Sugar: 1.3 grams
- Protein: 1.7 grams

Ingredients

- 12 hulled medium strawberries
- 2 ounces of quartered shortcakes
- ¼ cup of semi-sweet chocolate chips
- 1 tablespoon of margarine, low calorie

How to cook

1. Place a layer of waxed paper onto a cookie sheet.
2. Thread the strawberries and shortcakes alternately onto metal skewers.
3. In a small saucepan combine the margarine and chocolate chips and melt over low temperature.
4. Drizzle the chocolate over the kabobs, refrigerate for 4 minutes until set.

88. Raisin Oatmeal Spice Cookies
(Prep Time: 35 minutes/Serves: 36)

Smart points: 3

Nutritional Values Per Serving

- Calories: 61.1
- Saturated Fat: 4 grams
- Carbs: 13.2 gram
- Sugar: 0.8 grams
- Protein: 1.4 grams

Ingredients

- ¾ cups of brown sugar
- ½ a cup of sugar substitute
- ¾ cup of raisins
- 2 cups of rolled oats
- 1 cup of whole wheat flour
- 1 teaspoon of ground cinnamon
- ½ a teaspoon of ground nutmeg
- 1 teaspoon of baking soda
- 1 teaspoon of salt
- ¾ cup of unsweetened applesauce
- 1 egg
- 1 teaspoon of vanilla
- Cooking spray

How to cook

1. Preheat the oven to 395 degrees F.
2. Grease a baking large baking tray with cooking spray.
3. Combine the dry ingredients in a large bowl.

4. Add the vanilla, egg and applesauce and whisk together thoroughly.
5. Mold into walnut size balls and arrange on the baking tray.
6. Bake for 13 minutes until the edges are slightly browned.
7. Remove from the oven and allow to cool before serving.

89. Sunshine Fruit Pudding Salad
(Prep Time: 3 minutes/Serves: 6)

Smart points: 3

Nutritional Values Per Serving

- Calories: 94.3
- Saturated Fat: 0.3 grams
- Carbs: 24.3 gram
- Sugar: 2 grams
- Protein: 1 grams

Ingredients

- 1 can of mandarin oranges
- 1 can of pineapple chunks
- 1 can of instant vanilla pudding mix, fat free

How to cook

1. Combine all the ingredients including the juice from the canned fruit in a large bowl and stir to combine. Do not add water to the milk to the vanilla mix.
2. Chill for 1 hour before serving.

90. Banana Ice Cream
(Prep Time: 10 minutes/Serves: 2)

Smart points: 4

Nutritional Values Per Serving

- Calories: 120.8
- Saturated Fat: 0.9 grams
- Carbs: 27.9 grams
- Sugar: 3.1 grams
- Protein: 1.8 grams

Ingredients

- 2 ripe bananas, peeled, cut into chunks and frozen
- 2-4 tablespoons of milk or fruit juice
- 1 teaspoon of vanilla extract
- Sliced strawberries or chocolate syrup as a topping

How to cook

1. Blend the frozen bananas, vanilla extract and juice or milk into a puree.
2. Transfer into bowls and garnish with the topping of your choice.

Chapter 12 Drink Recipes

91. Champagne Raspberry Cocktail
(Prep Time: 5 minutes/Serves: 4)

Smart Points: 3

Nutritional Value Per Serving

- Calories: 99
- Saturated Fat: 0 grams
- Carbs: 10 grams
- Sugar: 2 gram
- Protein: 0 grams

Ingredients

- ¾ cup of chilled raspberry flavored juice
- 1 ½ cups of sparkling chilled wine
- 1 cup of chilled lemon seltzer
- Ice cubes
- ½ a cup of fresh raspberries
- 4 small mint sprigs

How to cook

1. Combine the seltzer, wine and juice in a pitcher.
2. Divide the ice into 4 wine glasses
3. Pour the cocktail mixture into the glasses
4. Garnish with the mint sprig and raspberry

92. Celery, Apple, Cucumber Juice
(Prep Time: 10 minutes/Serves: 2)

Smart Points: 2

Nutritional Value Per Serving

- Calories: 76
- Saturated Fat: 0 grams
- Carbs: 2 grams
- Sugar: 2 gram
- Protein: 3 grams

Ingredients

- 3 apples cored and quartered
- 2 peeled oranges
- 3 stalks of celery
- 1 peeled cucumber
- 1 handful of parsley
- ½ a peeled lemon
- 1 inch piece of fresh ginger
- Ice cubes

How to cook

1. Divide the ice into glasses
2. Put all the ingredients into a juicer and juice.
3. Pour over the ice and serve.

93. Green Iron Juice
(Prep Time: 10 minutes/Serves: 2)

Smart Points: 2

Nutritional Values Per Serving

- Calories: 86
- Saturated Fat: 0.8 grams
- Carbs: 8 grams
- Sugar: 2 grams
- Protein: 12 grams

Ingredients

- ½ a bunch of broccoli
- 1 handful of spinach
- ½ a cucumber
- 1 pear
- 1 peeled tangelo
- 1 peeled lemon
- 1 peeled lime
- 1 inch piece of peeled root ginger
- Ice cubes

How to cook

1. Wash the fruit and vegetables, chop them up and juice.
2. Divide the ice into cups, pour the juice over the top and serve.

94. Cucumber Kale and Pineapple Juice
(Prep Time: 10 minutes/Serves: 2)

Smart Points: 3

Nutritional Values Per Serving

- Calories: 85
- Saturated Fat: 0.6 grams
- Carbs: 10 grams
- Sugar: 3 grams
- Protein 2 grams

Ingredients

- 5 kale leaves
- ½ a large peeled cucumber
- ½ a bunch of cilantro
- ¼ of a peeled pineapple
- 1 green apple, sliced into quarters and cored
- Ice cubes

How to cook

1. Wash the fruit and chop it into pieces.
2. Put the chopped pieces into the juicer.
3. Divide the ice between glasses.
4. Pour the juice over the top and serve.

95. Date Coconut Smoothie
(Prep Time: 5 minutes/Serves: 2)

Smart Points: 3

Nutritional Values Per Serving

- Calories: 106
- Saturated Fat: 2.1 grams
- Carbs: 30.6 grams
- Sugar: 2.6 grams
- Protein: 12 grams

Ingredients

- 1 cup of coconut milk, unsweetened
- 1 banana
- 4 dates chopped and pitted
- 2 teaspoons of Nutella
- 1 cup of ice

How to cook

1. Blend the dates, banana and coconut milk in a food processor.
2. Add the ice and the Nutella and continue to blend.
3. Pour into glasses and serve.

96. Peach Blueberry Protein Shake
(Prep Time: 5 minutes/Serves: 1 serving)

Smart Points: 3

Nutritional Values Per Serving

- Calories: 134
- Saturated Fat: 3.0 grams
- Carbs: 9.2 grams
- Sugar: 2.5 grams
- Protein: 18.4 grams

Ingredients

- 1/3 cup of non fat cottage cheese
- 2 tablespoons of vanilla protein powder
- ¼ cup of blueberries
- ½ a cup of frozen peach slices
- ¼ cup of water
- Ice cubes
- Sweetener of your choice

How to cook

1. Add all of the ingredients to a food processer and blend until creamy and smooth.
2. Pour into a glass and serve.

97. Carrot Cake Smoothie
(Prep Time: 5 minutes/Serves: 1 serving)

Smart Points: 8

Nutritional Values Per Serving

- Calories: 288
- Saturated Fat: 3.7 grams
- Carbs: 32 grams
- Sugar: 7.4 grams
- Protein: 25 grams

Ingredients

- ½ a cup of low fat cottage cheese
- 1 scoop of protein powder, vanilla flavor
- ½ a cup of chopped carrots
- ½ a cup of pineapple, crushed with the juice
- 1 tablespoon of ground flaxseed
- ½ a teaspoon of ground cinnamon
- Ice cubes

How to cook

1. Place all of the ingredients into a food processor and blend until creamy and smooth.
2. Pour into glasses and serve.

98. Agua Watermelon Fresca
(Prep Time: 5 minutes/Serves: 4)

Smart Points: 2

Nutritional Values Per Serving

- Calories: 57
- Saturated Fat: 0 grams
- Carbs: 14 grams
- Sugar: 1 gram
- Protein: 1 gram

Ingredients

- 4 cups of seedless, cubed ripe sweet watermelon
- 1 ½ cups of water
- 1 tablespoon of honey
- 3 cups of water
- 3 tablespoons of fresh lime juice
- Fresh mint for garnish
- Ice

How to cook

1. Blend the watermelon, lime juice, honey and water until smooth.
2. Strain into a bowl.
3. Add the rest of the water and stir.
4. Refrigerate for 2 hours.
5. Divide ice into glasses, pour the chilled drink over the top, garnish with mint

99. Pina Colada
(Prep Time: 5 minutes/Serves:1 serving)

Smart Points: 5

Nutritional Values Per Serving

- Calories: 183
- Saturated Fat: 0.5 grams
- Carbs: 11 grams
- Sugar: 0.5 grams
- Protein: 9.5 grams

Ingredients

- 3 tablespoons of natural vanilla protein powder
- ¼ cup of crushed pineapple with juice
- 1 ½ ounces of white rum
- 1/8 teaspoon of coconut extract
- 1 cup of ice

How to cook

1. Blend the ingredients in a food processor.
2. Pour into glasses and serve.

100. Banana Peanut Butter Chocolate Shake
(Prep Time: 5 minutes/Serves: 1 serving)

Smart Points: 8

Nutritional Values Per Serving

- Calories: 299
- Saturated Fat: 6.1 grams
- Carbs: 29.6 grams
- Sugar: 5.9 grams
- Protein: 36.2 grams

Ingredients

- ½ a cup of non fat cottage cheese
- 2 tablespoons of peanut butter flour
- 1 scoop of chocolate protein powder
- ½ a frozen banana
- 1 cup of ice
- 1 teaspoon of honey

How to cook

1. Blend all the ingredients in a food processor until smooth.
2. Pour into glasses and serve.

Conclusion

I hope this book was able to inform you on the basics of Weight Loss Freestyle, the organization's goals, and its methodology to help participants lose weight.

The next step is to start preparing healthy and nutritious meals for your breakfast, lunch, and dinner. This can be a daunting step, but you have a recipe book full of quick and easy choices. Start with recipes that are a variation on something you already know how to cook and work from there. With a little bit of effort you won't even need to refer to this book to come up with a quick healthy meal for any time of day.

If you do not want to start your weight loss journey alone, consider looking into attending meetings at your local Weight Loss Freestyle. Here you will find support from people that have the same goal you do – it's a great place to go and share experiences about weight loss.

Thank you and good luck!

Appendix Table of Smart Point Value

For you to have an idea of how many Smart Points are assigned to a particular food item, here is a list of the most common food items that are eaten by a majority of Weight Watchers members. Take note that the Smart Point allocation to each food item is dependent on the number of calories and the level of fat content.

¼ avocado (2 Smart Points)

¼ cup of almonds (4 Smart Points)

1 cup of brown rice (6 Smart Points)

1 cup of cottage cheese (2 Smart Points)

1 cup of 2% reduced fat milk (5 Smart Points)

1 cup of cooked oatmeal (5 Smart Points)

1 cup of low-fat milk (4 Smart Points)

1 cup of plain almond milk (1 Smart Point)

1 cup of skim milk (3 Smart Points)

1 cup of sugarless black coffee (0 Smart Points)

1 egg (2 Smart Points)

1 egg white (0 Smart Points)

1 fried egg (3 Smart Points)

1 ounce of crumbled feta (3 Smart Points)

1 ounce of tortilla chips (4 Smart Points)

1 slice of American cheese (4Smart Points)

1 slice of bread (2 Smart Points)

1 tablespoon of butter (5 Smart Points)

1 tablespoon of honey (4 Smart Points)

1 tablespoon of mayonnaise (3 Smart Points)

1 tablespoon of olive oil (4 Smart Points)

1 teaspoon of sugar (1 Smart Points)

2 ounces of sliced deli turkey (1 Smart Points)

2 tablespoons of fat-free half and a half (1 Smart Points)

2 tablespoons of peanut butter (6 Smart Points)

2 tablespoons of ranch salad dressing (5 Smart Points)

3 ounces of cooked shrimp (1 Smart Point)

3 ounces of ground beef (4 Smart Points)

3 slices of cooked bacon (5 Smart Points)

5 ounces of red wine (4 Smart Points)

5 ounces of white wine (4 Smart Points)

Any bagel (5 Smart Points)

Apple (0 Smart Points)

Asparagus (0 Smart Points)

Baby carrots (0 Smart Points)

Banana (0 Smart Points)

Berries, mixed (0 Smart Points)

Blackberries (0 Smart Points)

Blueberries (0 Smart Points)

Broccoli (0 Smart Points)

Canned black beans (3 Smart Points)

Canned tuna fish ounces (1 Smart Point)

Cantaloupe (0 Smart Points)

Carrots (0 Smart Points)

Celery (0 Smart Points)

Cheddar cheese (4 Smart Points)

Cherries (0 Smart Points)

Cherry tomatoes (0 Smart Points)

Chicken breast (2 Smart Points)

Cooked sweet potatoes (3 Smart Points)

Cooked turkey bacon (3 Smart Points)

Corn on the cob (4 Smart Points)

Cucumber (0 Smart Points)

Diet Coke (0 Smart Points)

English muffin (4 Smart Points)

Fat-free salsa (0 Smart Points)

French fries (13 Smart Points)

Fresh fruit (0 Smart Points)

Grape tomatoes (0 Smart Points)

Grapefruit (0 Smart Points)

Grapes (0 Smart Points)

Green beans (0 Smart Points)

Guacamole (1 Smart Points)

Hamburger bun (5 Smart Points)

Homemade chocolate chip cookies (3 Smart Points)

Hummus, two tablespoons (2 Smart Points)

Italian salad dressing (3 Smart Points)

Lettuce (0 Smart Points)

Luncheon meat (2 Smart Points)

Mango (0 Smart Points)

Mashed potatoes (4 Smart Points)

Mixed greens salad (0 Smart Points)

Mushrooms (0 Smart Points)

Mustard, one tablespoon (0 Smart Points)

Nectarine (0 Smart Points)

Once ounce of coly cheese (4 Smart Points)

Onions (0 Smart Points)

Orange (0 Smart Points)

Peach (0 Smart Points)

Pear (0 Smart Points)

Pineapple (0 Smart Points)

Plain baked potatoes (5 Smart Points)

Plain Greek yogurt (3 Smart Points)

Pork Chop (3 Smart Points)

Raspberries (0 Smart Points)

Regular beer (5 Smart Points)

Regular pasta (5 Smart Points)

Salad dressing, or balsamic vinaigrette (1 Smart Points)

Scrambled eggs with milk and butter (6 Smart Points)

Spinach (0 Smart Points)

Strawberries (0 Smart Points)

Sweet red peppers (0 Smart Points)

Tomatoes (0 Smart Points)

Tortilla, flour (3 Smart Points)

Two tablespoons of half and half cream (2 Smart Points)

Water (0 Smart Points)

Watermelon (0 Smart Points)

White rice, cooked, 1 cup (6 Smart Points)

Whole milk (7 Smart Points)

Zucchini (0 Smart Points)

Made in the USA
Middletown, DE
08 August 2018